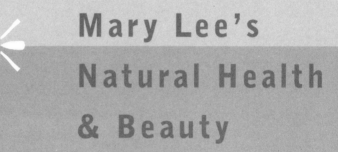

Mary Lee's
Natural Health
& Beauty

Mary Lee Patton

with Bob Condor

JEREMY P. TARCHER / PUTNAM
A MEMBER OF
PENGUIN PUTNAM INC.
NEW YORK

Mary Lee's

Natural Health & Beauty

Healthy Living with Essential Oils

This book is not intended to prescribe or diagnose. In no way do the authors intend to replace any medical health practitioner. For serious medical conditions, the authors encourage the consultation of a physician.

Most Tarcher/Putnam books are available at special quantity discounts for bulk purchases for sales promotions, premiums, fund-raising, and educational needs. Special books or book excerpts also can be created to fit specific needs. For details, write or telephone Putnam Special Markets, 375 Hudson Street, New York, NY 10014.

Jeremy P. Tarcher/Putnam
a member of
Penguin Putnam Inc.
375 Hudson Street
New York, NY 10014
www.penguinputnam.com

Library of Congress Cataloging-in-Publication Data

Patton, Mary Lee, date.
    Mary Lee's natural health & beauty : healthy living with essential oils /
Mary Lee Patton, with Bob Condor.
        p.   cm.
    Includes bibliographical references.
    ISBN 1-58542-105-7
    1. Beauty, Personal.   2. Essences and essential oils.
3. Herbal cosmetics.   4. Aromatherapy.   5. Women—Health and hygiene.
I. Title: Mary Lee's natural health and beauty.   II. Title: Natural health & beauty.
III. Condor, Bob.   IV. Title.
RA778.P297   2001
613'.04244—dc21   00-066766

Printed in the United States of America

10   9   8   7   6   5   4   3   2   1

This book is printed on acid-free paper. ∞

Book design by Lovedog Studio

This book is more important to your family's health than any other you will read this year.

Mary Lee Patton offers clear, scientifically based advice about the chemicals in products we use every day in our homes and with our children. She talks about everything from choosing better shampoos, oils, and soaps for our kids to getting healthier skin for ourselves.

I am the pediatrician for Mary Lee's two sons, and I have watched the results of her awareness in them. I have also been asked hundreds of questions over the years about the chemicals in cleaning solutions and personal care products. All too often, my answer about medical knowledge of long-term toxicity has to be, "We don't know." That answer alone is enough to convince me that we have to do much more to find answers. Meanwhile, we can look for safer, toxin-free soaps, shampoos, and other household products.

There are safe, effective treatments for many problems that we doctors have been trained to ignore. Mary Lee's book takes a positive approach to health, and she uses solutions with safety records that date back centuries.

This book has useful information for parents, kids, and everyone else. Doctors could learn a lot, too. . . .

—Jay Gordon, M.D.
Fellow, American Academy of Pediatrics

Acknowledgments

For me, one thing has been clear since early childhood: My life's mission is and always will be to guide people in the return to a natural way of living.

Ralph Waldo Emerson, the great American poet and essayist, once wrote, "Our chief want in life is somebody who shall make us do what we can." I have been blessed to have several of those special somebodies in my life, helping me fulfill my mission:

My husband, Jim, who taught me how to be a warrior, and to keep working for what I believe in, no matter how the odds are stacked.

My dearest loves, my twin boys, Micah and Talor. You have always shared Mommy with her work, and I thank you for letting it be a part of our lives. Each night when I tuck you in and see those bright eyes and smiling faces, I know why I do what I do.

My partner, Bob Condor, whom I want to acknowledge for his kindness, brilliance, balance, and immense talent. Again the stars were shining on me when my agents, Frank Weimann and Frank Coffey, asked Bob to join me on this project. He turned my volumes of rough scribblings and research into flowing paragraphs and chapters that speak beautifully. More than just a great writer, Bob is a loving father and husband who truly lives what he writes about.

I thank Frank Weimann and Frank Coffey at the Literary Group for giving me this opportunity and finding the right team to bring it to fruition. And what a team: Hillery Borton, our editor, brought enthusiasm, smarts, and a wholehearted belief that this book is right on, and right on time; and without our publicist, Ken Siman, and his hard work, experience, and the respect he has among his industry peers, this book would never have taken the giant steps it did. Thank you also, Kelly Groves!

To my associates at Earth Tribe, too numerous to mention, I thank you for your tremendous support. And to my girlfriends Mara, Heidi, and Char, who were with me on that fateful day when I blew up the oven, thanks for staying close through the years and through the miles.

To my sister Jean, the true writer in the family, your love and gift for writing have amazed me since we were little; my sister Joey, my biggest supporter, thank you for believing; and my little brother Bobby, thanks for spending endless hours patiently exploring the woods with me.

Thank you to my mother and father, and my grandmothers and grandfathers, who triumphed over and struggled under Mother Nature. I especially thank you, Mom and Dad, for staying there and raising us in the North Woods.

—Mary Lee

Writing a book involves the ongoing dance of individuality and teamwork. This project was no exception. As coauthors, Mary Lee and I started the project as strangers but quickly forged our partnership on a common goal: Persuade people to get chemicals out of their lives.

I learned so much from Mary Lee about how essential oils of plants can replace chemicals effectively in all parts of daily life—from feeling more energetic to cleaning the house to shampooing my hair (and those precious young scalps of Artie and Lana). It is my privilege to help her give voice to a vital message. Topping that, it is my fortune to share Mary Lee's inspirational life story with you, one that pivoted on a personal tragedy that she turned into a lifelong commitment to help others.

While working, Mary Lee and I talked a lot about what mattered most to us—our spouses, kids, family, and friends. Our connection to loved ones seemed to give the book a special boost of energy, like so many drops of rosemary essential oil, when we needed them most.

We realized this book was about more than introducing essential oils as an effective and naturally healthy alternative. The bigger message was how to make life better for the people we love the most. It made the late nights, early mornings, and disrupted weekends more tolerable.

I am fortunate to have the ongoing support and wisdom of my editors at the *Chicago Tribune,* including Howard Tyner, Ann Marie Lipinski, Gerry Kern, Geoff Brown, Janet Franz, Denise Joyce, Ross Werland, and Wendy Navratil. It is my honor to work for them and the newspaper.

I profoundly benefit from the insight and friendship of my mentor, Tom Emmerson. I spent a good part of two months with him on the

Iowa State University campus in the throes of this project. He taught me long ago to be myself, that it was the straightest line to my dreams.

My thanks to Frank Weimann and Frank Coffey at The Literary Group for envisioning Mary Lee and me as partners. Frank Coffey, in particular, probably lost count of the phone hours spent during the proposal phase of this project.

This book gained immensely from the guidance of our editor at Tarcher/Putnam, Hillery Borton. Her enthusiasm was relentless and she provided just the kinds of good ideas writers can only hope to receive. We also feel indebted to our copy editor, Paulette McGee, for her keen eye. We are grateful for the hard work of our publicist, Ken Siman, plus everyone at Tarcher/Putnam who believed in the potential of this book.

Of course, the dance between individuality and teamwork is no more apparent than in a writer's own home and family. My deepest inspiration comes from my soulmate and wife, Mary. I am in constant awe of her spirit and verve and unmatchable curiosity. We refused to let this book detour our journey with our children, Arthur and Lana, who both had third birthdays during the writing phase of this project.

But too many times I jumped back on the computer after the kids were in bed. Nonetheless, Mary was always there with fresh ideas, excellent questions, and a gentle arm on my back or neck when I seemed to need it most. There is simply no one in the world like her. I cherish every minute we have together. I will always save the last dance for her—and only her.

—Bob Condor

For my boys, my muses,
Micah and Talor,
who inspire me each day to dream

—M.L.

For Mary, Arthur, and Lana,
who grace my every day
with an abundance
of natural beauty

—B.C.

Contents

Chapter 9. Oils as Everyday Medicine

Essential oils can change your life—and *healthstyle*—for the better. Plant oils can unleash energy you didn't even know was inside you.

Chapter 10. Rethinking Skin and Beauty Care

Too many American women put too many synthetic chemicals on their faces, hair, hands, breasts, legs, you name it. Some government experts have estimated up to 200 chemicals a day!

Chapter 11. Detoxing Your Beauty Routine

A practical discussion about parts of the beauty regimen that occupy lots of time but not always with best results.

Safety Information

Appendix A: *Earth Tribe* Essential Oils and Products

Appendix B: Suggested Reading and Reference List

Introduction

My Story

I am still trying to figure out why we decided to bake omelets that day, rather than make them in a pan. Let's just agree it was a bad idea.

One Saturday morning during my college days at the University of Minnesota, I invited some girlfriends over for breakfast. A friend turned on the oven for me, but she didn't know it was an old-fashioned oven for which you had to light the pilot light each time you turned it on.

I didn't realize she had turned the gas dial to a high setting. So when I bent over to light the pilot with a burning match, the oven and our omelet-baking session literally blew up in my face. Flames curled and snapped upward, engulfing my face, hair, neck, and chest.

I was blown back several feet, or so my friends recall. I don't remember much except some awful smells of burned skin and hair.

My friends immediately called for an ambulance and thoughtfully tried to keep me away from my reflection while we waited. But I insisted on looking in the mirror to see how badly my face and body had been burned.

It was bad.

Really bad.

I went into shock by the time the paramedics arrived. I was devastated. I was twenty years old and had always been considered attractive. My sense of self changed in an instant.

At the hospital, the doctors X-rayed my chest to see if my lungs were burned. They were not, but the news did little to cheer me up. I had second-degree burns pretty much from my waist up on the front of my body. My face and neck got the worst of it, the skin bright red, raw, and peeling.

My friends were loving and spent endless hours by my side at the hospital. But I couldn't stop sobbing for five straight days.

One pal not at the omelet party visited me. My wounds had been dressed but were open to the air. She didn't recognize me at all, walking right by me and thinking I must in the other bed in the semiprivate room.

The chief resident physician in the burn unit came to see me about halfway through the hospital stay. This was the low point for me.

"Hmm, this doesn't look good," he said. "Not good at all."

He told me that I would likely have some permanent scarring and that it would take years for my skin to heal completely. He predicted that I would age prematurely and that staying out of the sun at all times would be critical. He said I could look ten to twenty years older than my peers.

The doctor left and I cried hard. As much as I wanted to be strong, I couldn't help feeling sorry for myself.

Then, like a sunrise that starts to fill the morning sky, I started talking to myself. I began to say, "I'm going to heal." At first, it was a fleeting thought, a glimmer of hope and light. Then I started to say it over and over. "I am going to heal. I am going to heal. I am going to heal."

Then I started to think, okay, how am I going to heal?

The answer came to me from my past. I would use plants on my face, just as I had been taught as a child by family members when I was growing up in northern Minnesota. I would seek out the right healing herbs and essential oils I was studying in classes I had been taking at local health food stores in Minneapolis. I would pull out my old copies of *East-West Journal* and *Mother Jones* magazines. I would think positive. I would show that doctor he was wrong. I would heal.

My first stop once I was released from the hospital was to visit an herbalist I knew in the West Bank of Minneapolis. He recommended lavender oil and aloe vera. He showed me how to make a gel for my face, neck, arms, and chest. Then he added a critical element: put a few drops of lavender oil on my pillowcase at night. "It will keep your spirits up," he said.

I went straight home and put the gel all over my burns. I applied more before going to bed.

The next morning, before even looking in the mirror, I knew I was healing. Then I looked in the mirror. My skin was less red and peeling.

Every morning for the next week, I couldn't wait to look in the mirror, even though I knew before one peek that my skin was restoring itself.

The lavender drops on my pillowcase may have been even more important. Illnesses and injuries can hurt our souls even more than our bodies. I believe the lavender kept me upright when self-pity could easily have brought me down; amazingly, I didn't even need to take any of the painkillers prescribed by my doctors at the hospital.

At the end of the week, one of my girlfriends wanted to take me to the university spring carnival. She knew I hadn't been out much since leaving the hospital and thought the event might get my mind off the accident. When she came to my apartment, and when I opened the door, she couldn't believe her eyes! My face looked so much better that she burst into tears, and so did I, this time for joy. I tied a scarf around my neck, which was still a bit red and raw, and went to the carnival with confidence. We skipped practically the whole way there.

I visited the chief resident at the hospital the next day. He was practically speechless. "I don't believe what I am seeing," he said.

The doctor then called several colleagues in to take a look and none of them could believe it. Certainly none of them were convinced that essential oil from lavender flowers and extracted juice from the aloe vera plant, along with positive thinking, were the healing agents.

But I knew it and that was enough, at least for a start. I could literally look at myself in the mirror and see proof that essential plant oils and the human mind make for a potent and healing combination. I had healed without any scars. The next step was to let the world know it.

That was twenty years ago, and since then I have devoted my life to studying essential plant oils and finding ways to help people use them in their everyday lives. My mission is simple: Show people how to use essential plant oils in their everyday lives so they can reconnect with nature, resurrect a powerful way of healing, and be more fully alive.

My Healthy Living plan is not about making some radical set of changes in your everyday world. It won't ask you to stop using your cell phone (I have one), abandon your busy schedule, or never enjoy your favorite foods. Rather, I will encourage you to take small, easy steps, one at a time, to build a sort of "natural momentum" in your health and beauty regimens. What you do with your newfound energy and zest for living is your choice. Essential plant oils will make it possible to change your life without changing your lifestyle.

It is our time to reclaim what this good Earth has offered our families and community for so long. That's why I named my company *Earth Tribe*. We all have the common privilege of the grass under our feet, flowers in the garden or window, trees that provide shade, and natural fresh air. Most of all, we can share in the healing properties of plants and—get this—improve the environment at the same time. The purpose of this book is to show you how.

After the accident, I returned to my studies at the University of Minnesota and even did some modeling. Believe it or not, one of my teachers, an English professor, didn't accept that I had missed classes because I was burned on the face. He actually made me bring a note from my doctors at the university hospital.

It took about two months for me to completely heal from the burns, especially on my arms and chest. I stayed out of the sun as much as possible to help the process. While I was physically returning to my former self, I was changing inside. My spirit was emerging in an entirely new way, urging me to find my life's work and mission.

I felt compelled to study essential plant oils. I lobbied my professors to let me develop an independent study curriculum that would cover holistic medicine and healing practices, adding some outside courses to supplement what the university didn't offer. But they basically considered me foolish, and several of them figured there was no future in being a natural health practitioner. Of course, this was eighteen years ago and no universities were attuned to any sort of alternative healing methods. Wow, has that changed in a hurry! Now, Harvard physician and prominent researcher Dr. David Eisenberg says, three-quarters of all American medical schools currently offer courses in alternative medicine. But, back then, I found it impossible to formally study essential plant oils anywhere in the United States. Taking classes at the local health food stores would only go so far.

Fortunately for me, as this has developed into my life's work, I was dating a Swedish dentist at the time. He was offered a job with a pharmaceutical company in Sweden and I went with him. We lived in Athens, London, and Stockholm, where I excitedly took courses at every stop.

It was wonderful to study clinical aromatherapy, especially in Britain, where it was by then considered part of mainstream medicine. I learned the science behind essential oils—and, believe me, there is plenty of it—while getting a feel for what single-note oils or blends can help people heal illnesses or create more energy in their daily lives.

I studied with instructors who are now considered masters in essential oils and aromatherapy. I also worked for a European pharmaceutical company that was a leader in providing herbal products. The European market, especially Germany with its Commission E (equivalent to the U.S. Food and Drug Administration), is a good ten to twenty years ahead of us in understanding how herbs and other plants can be potent, effective medicines.

When I returned to the United States, I started making my own oils and products, such as soaps, shampoos, and household cleaners. The soaps, in particular, reminded me of my own childhood. I lived on the Leech Lake Indian Reservation in northern Minnesota. We attended the weekly pow-wow on Thursday nights. My great-grandmother and grandmother had used wild plants to cure any ills, boiling mushrooms, pulling up one root or another on our property or making poultices of onion and mint leaves for colds. Grandma regularly put up a batch of soaps with peppermint and spearmint oils. They were ugly little soaps— the kind you now see in the most fashionable boutiques! To me, they didn't look unsightly until I visited my school friends' homes in Walker, Minnesota. Their bathroom soap dishes held washable Cupids and hearts. What I knew then was that they were much prettier than our soaps at home. What I know now is that these soaps were filled with chemicals and fillers and other artificial ingredients. Chapters 10 and 11 of this book will discuss typical mass-produced American beauty and personal hygiene products containing chemicals. It's time for all of us to rethink how we use products with chemicals in our homes—for the sake of our families and our environment.

At first, I had no intention of starting a business. While working as a flight attendant, I fell in love with Los Angeles and southern California during layovers, so I moved there. Over the next few years, I was simply blending oils and making products for myself and friends. I would combine different oils for skin care, colds and flu, first aid, and premenstrual syndrome. Everybody loved them and more than a few people suggested I should market the products.

One friend was so enthusiastic she set up a lunchtime seminar for me at the Beverly Wilshire Hotel in 1992. It turned out several beauty editors from national women's magazines were in attendance. I was pregnant with my twin boys, Micah and Taylor, who are now eight years old. I talked about plant oils and let everyone sample some of my "products."

Woman's Day magazine ran an item about the seminar and my "company" in its "Editor's Choice" column, mentioning my P.O. box address (I didn't even have a toll-free telephone number). The babies were born by the time it was published—they were maybe two or three months old—so I was obviously quite busy with them. One of my newest projects was developing oils that I could use in caring for them from infancy through their entire childhood and adult years.

One day, weeks after the item ran, I stopped by my mailbox. It was overflowing with envelopes. There was note saying, "Please come to the window for more mail!" The postal clerk hefted a huge box of letters— all inquiries about the *Woman's Day* piece on aromatherapy and essential oils.

I took the letters home, grinning to myself, completely in shock. Friends and family members urged me to start a business.

I was more than a little intrigued. The burn accident and my healing made me always want to educate people about the power of essential oils and plants. Developing a home-based business was an ideal match for my goal of wanting to be with the twins as much as possible. Plus, I had discovered so many new uses for oils during pregnancy—which I will cover in detail—including blending lavender, chamomile, grapeseed, and wheat germ oils to eliminate stretch marks, and using oils to help raise healthy children (an ongoing passion and project of mine).

I thought back to my own childhood when my mother joked that I was a witch doctor because I was always taking in sick birds and nursing them back to health with my own potions. I gradually moved to injured bunnies, geese, dogs, cats, and even my horses (cats especially because it made me feel like the girl in *The Three Lives of Thomasina,* whose cat came back to life). I guess healing is in my blood and heritage.

One day my husband, Jim, and I were discussing the possibility of starting a business. Jim said, "You won't help many people if only a few people know about your products. If you believe in essential oils and natural products so strongly, you need to get the message to as many people as you can."

That single statement hit me squarely in the heart and soul. It was my epiphany. I knew my mission was clear. I would bring my message to people through my business. *Earth Tribe* would be my vehicle for spreading my message of physical, emotional, and spiritual healing. I wanted to show the world how to live a simple, more natural and chemical-free life every day. Even if it meant that in the beginning I would make my own *Earth Tribe* labels in late-night sessions at the print shop and hire a nanny, Sylvia, who alternated holding babies and pouring oils into individual product bottles. What helped a lot was moving into a new house with a separate area where I could set up an office and "lab." I wasn't a twenty-something flight attendant blending oils in my kitchen anymore. Jim helped me set up educational seminars every Wednesday night and

Earth Healing

Colleen Anderson

Probably one of the most inviting things about plant oils, at least from my perspective, is that they bring feminine healing to the forefront. I have seen *Earth Tribe* oils bring women's wisdom back to families and communities.

For instance, one California woman, Colleen Anderson, noticed the cubbyholes at her daughter's kindergarten classroom were infested with ants. Since this is where the kids kept their lunches, Colleen decided to speak to the teacher about it. The teacher expressed little concern because she seemed to think the ants only appeared after lunch. Colleen didn't push the issue, but told the teacher she knew a nontoxic way to gently discourage the ants from coming into the classroom, and if she was interested to let her know.

The next morning Colleen was greeted at the door by her daughter's teacher, who had found ants in the cubbyholes and wondered if

(continued)

Saturday morning; I invited any friends or acquaintances who were interested in helping sell my products to act as "sales consultants."

The business started growing. We seem to keep expanding our offices and laboratory in Santa Monica, though I still make sure every batch of oils is handcrafted. Some 700 people are sales consultants, and we train some of them to train new consultants in the *Earth Tribe* mission and approach. Of course, I still believe in being a mommy to my boys.

I think essential oils and aromatherapy are the most important "rediscovery" of our times. Plant oils reconnect us with nature and, in the process, we can begin healing centuries of human disconnection from nature and decades of industrialized destruction of the environment.

For example, using essential oils can bring a family together. Jim and I started the ritual of using aromatherapy massage whenever someone in the house is sick. We all take turns applying oils to whoever is feeling the effects of a cold or flu, most typically on the temples, neck, breastbone, and upper shoulders. The boys love it, so do we, and we are strengthening the healing bond of touch between us.

What's more, plant oils awaken our sense of smell. Cutting-edge research is showing that our olfactory sense is about much more than pleasant smells and aromas. Plant oils can significantly impact the brain, whether it is to sharpen memory, ease depression, or increase creativity.

Earth Healing (continued)

Colleen could take care of them. Colleen had her *Earth Tribe* peppermint essential oil and *Earth Tribe All Natural Insect Repellant* with her. She asked for a bucket of warm water and added the peppermint oil. She threw in a bunch of clean sponges and rounded up the kids to help her wash away the ants. The peppermint oil works by washing away the scented trail that the ants leave to get to the food, and leaving a peppermint-scented trail, which the ants do *not* like.

The kids had a great time, and it was wonderful to know that this was something totally natural and nontoxic. Colleen finished the cleanup by spraying *Earth Tribe All Natural Insect Repellant* blend along what seemed to be the ants' entry points. Months later, the cubbyholes were still free of ants.

I believe that if you follow your heart, doors will open where you don't even know there are doors. You can almost feel the rush of fresh air on your face. This is so important for all of us, and especially women, to understand. If making money is your only goal or objective, it gets in the way, holds you back from your true prosperity—sort of like a wall. If you don't think about the money, or at least don't let it dominate your thoughts and actions, but keep to what you love, to what helps people, then the profits will come. It will almost be effortless.

I did say "almost." Make no mistake, sticking to your mission can be hard work. But if you believe in your core purpose—I think constantly about how I can make the world a better and more livable place for the next generation, which my boys personify to me—then you will find a way through the difficult times. Doing good leads to feeling good, and it starts with you and the people you love most.

These days, when I get the mail or sign onto our Internet site (www.earth-tribe.com), I have the privilege of reading testimonials and personal letters about our products from customers. It certainly gives me reason to keep going and spreading the message about essential oils. I remember one day reading a letter while standing in line at the bank. Tears were running down my face as I absorbed the words of a woman who said she was suicidal after a terrible auto accident. She explained that she was allergic to most medications that might help her mental state. Instead, she used our *Calming* product. She said it strengthened her spirit when her body felt too weak to even stand, that it cleared her mind when fog was the only thing in her forecast for weeks. I could barely catch my breath, thinking about a college girl and the plan to bake omelets. I had discovered the power of essential oils, the healing and sacredness and energy it can bring to everyday living, and now so had this woman. I felt honored to have contributed somehow to her quality of life.

This book is my chance to keep spreading the word, helping people to stand up for themselves, their families, and what they believe in. I hope you can use this book to find your own voice in a world that needs every last one.

Consider this Healthy Living plan to be your own, sort of a trusted companion at your side. Plant oils can change lives, one body, one mind, one soul at a time.

Chapter 1

Good from the First Drop

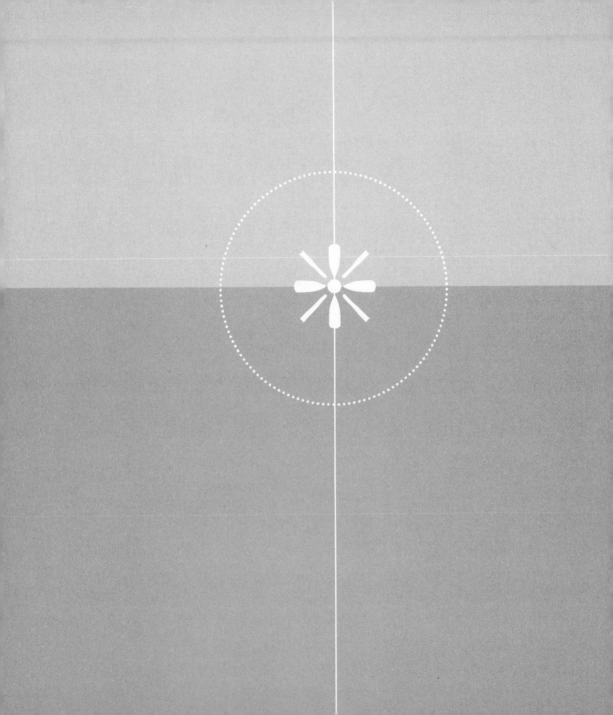

The best healthy living plan builds on itself. You take a first step and then keep moving forward. One good health habit leads to another, then another, and another. A personal momentum builds and inspires you to keep making healthy changes. Soon enough you start feeling positive about yourself.

That's how my Healthy Living plan starts. I will not ask you to go on some strict diet (the typical American woman will try twenty of them over a lifetime) or buy a health club membership (rationalizing that the cost will motivate you enough to work out).

Aromatherapy and essential plant oils can change your life precisely because you don't count fat grams or try to cram another activity into your day. To begin with, all you have to do is find room for several drops of lavender oil. You can run a bath and use about eight to ten drops in the water, then soak for at least ten minutes (take an extra ten, it will feel glorious and energizing and liberating all at the same time!). Or you can add a few drops to a wet washcloth in the shower; reapply once if you're in the shower long enough.

That is step one in its entirety. Pretty simple, right?

After one week, you will begin to feel the difference. Among other sensations you are likely to feel more revitalized and clear-headed after bathing. If you use the bath or shower at night, this step will improve your sleep. These are subtle changes, but they are not to be underestimated—every day with lavender increases self-awareness. I see the results with my clients and *Earth Tribe* customers. In two to three weeks, their skin glows and their energy is up.

They feel more physically alive, wake up more refreshed, drink less coffee, and sleep more soundly. Many people tell me their emotions feel more balanced and they are better able to focus their attention. Once these effects take hold we can move into a more comprehensive healing system to help such problems as adult acne, colds and flu, hormonal flux, or fatigue.

The therapeutic benefits of the lavender itself are part of such positive changes, but we'll get to that. There is another phenomenon at work here. Call it *addition by subtraction*. By eliminating soap products that contain synthetic chemicals and fragrances, you will be sparing your body the harsh effects of artificial washing. It might be influencing more than you think or will ever know.

And don't be fooled by soaps and other toiletries that claim to be natural. I have seen shelves of so-called citrus-based skin care products in health stores that don't have a single drop of juice from a lemon, orange, tangerine, or grapefruit—not to mention containing no pure essential oils. The citrus is as synthetic as wax fruit.

In its pure form, lavender is potent enough to do the job but mild enough to not overdo it. Your skin benefits, of course, but remember the skin is an entry point to your bloodstream and major organs.

Why start with lavender? Because it is the most gentle and versatile plant oil. It is excellent in the bath for adults and kids, even babies (use three to eight drops for kids depending on their age and size). The purple-flowered plant contains substances called coumarins that have been documented in lab studies to induce a calming effect on the body. For instance, research shows that when individuals smell lavender, that alpha brain waves are increased. These brain waves are associated with relaxation and stress reduction.

Lavender is nontoxic and experts believe it is effective when applied to the skin and works just as well when inhaled into the respiratory tract. The solar plexus—the area between the chest and stomach—is recommended as the best place to apply a few drops for calming effect. The soles of the feet are another good spot. You can mix it with sweet almond oil for a spine massage, which is quite soothing for infants. *Earth Tribe* makes a patented *Calming* blend that contains lavender and chamomile for maximum relief of both physical and emotional anxiety.

Moms and dads, take note. Philippe Mailhebiau, the French scientist and author of a widely respected set of monographs on essential oils, says lavender is good for children who are "stressed and disturbed by things going badly within the family environment."

A study in the British medical journal *The Lancet* showed that inhaling the scent of lavender induced sleep as effectively as medications—and without the side effects. Lavender prepares you for sleep but does not cause drowsiness. Over-the-counter sleep remedies can cause a sort of hangover effect the next morning. Other studies show how lavender, when applied to the temples or inhaled, relaxes blood vessels that can cause headaches.

What's more, you can use lavender for blemishes, burns, rashes, cuts, scrapes, general skin care, sunburn, and dandruff. That's one reason why some natural health practitioners call it the "Swiss Army knife" of herbs.

Many European doctors and aromatherapists are perhaps most impressed by lavender's natural ability to regenerate the skin. There is no synthetic medication or salve that can match it. I can certainly attest to that; it heals skin rapidly and without scarring.

Other physicians and researchers are even more enthused about lavender as a natural antibiotic—without the side effects of kidney toxicity, anemia, or lowered white cell count. Lavender provides protection against infections without any threat of a super bacteria reaction, which has been occurring with synthetic medications, forcing drug makers to develop more and more potent medications. Another plus, lavender doesn't destroy the "good" bacteria, or flora, in the stomach and intestinal tract that actually fights off infections. Again, the herb does its job without overdoing it.

Academic research indicates that lavender works similarly to antibiotic drugs. Cornell University researchers have demonstrated its potential for killing certain kinds of staph infections, while many aromatherapists have seen the results of lavender for reducing the frequency and intensity of both the common cold and flu viruses. Strange as it might seem—though it's less strange than it may have seemed even three years ago—there are health practitioners who believe lavender will be one of our most effective medicines of the new millennium.

Best of all, lavender reconnects us to nature and ancient healing traditions. Lavender comes from the word *lavare,* which means "to wash" in Latin. Lavender flowers and leaves were used to perfume baths and give the water in which people washed a pleasant smell during the days of early Greek, Roman, and Persian civilizations. I'm sure they found that lavender is a disinfectant, as well as being aromatic. It was also tucked into linens to make them smell fresh. You can even find references to this in the Bible.

In the Middle Ages lavender was used to embalm corpses, cure animals of lice, and repel mosquitoes. In France, people noted that glove manufacturers who scented their goods with lavender were less likely to catch the bubonic plague, prompting widespread use of the herb to ward off illness for centuries. It was regularly used in sickrooms and to boost patients' spirits; lavender water was spritzed on bedclothes and pillows. During Victorian times, lavender oil was used as an ingredient in smelling salts to help people with fainting spells. During World Wars I and II, English doctors used the plant oil as antiseptic when surgical supplies ran low.

Lavender's powers might be as spiritual as they are therapeutic. In Tuscany, a sprig of freshly picked lavender is boiled in water and then a child is washed in the water to remove the child's so-called "evil eye"— believed to have the power to harm others. Lavender has long been considered the herb of love and peace.

Throughout Europe and parts of Asia, lavender is still a health and wellness staple. It is used in syrups and lozenges to soothe coughs and

You will learn more about how to use essential oils throughout this book. For starters, here are some therapeutic applications for lavender and other oils. Some of the identified oils and products are in our *Earth Tribe* line; see Appendix A for details and ingredients.

INHALATION

- Inhale directly from bottle.
- Wear on pulse points as a perfume.
- Place a few drops on a piece of cotton or handkerchief and carry it with you.
- To calm children at night, place two or three drops of lavender on their pillow-case.

DIFFUSION

- Place in a diffuser lightbulb ring, which is sold by aromatherapy/essential oil companies and natural health stores.
- Place in aromatherapy clay pots.
- Use an electric nebulizing diffuser for larger spaces.
- Spray into the air (mix with *Earth Tribe Base Spray* to scent a room).
- Place a few drops into a humidifier or vaporizer during cold and flu season as a preventive measure.

BODY AND FOOT BATHS

- For a refreshing foot bath, place five to seven drops of your favorite essential oil into a warm bath or a tub of warm water. We suggest *Detox, Energize,* or *Breathe.*

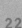

- One of the best methods for getting the most out of essential oils is a full body bath. After you have run a bath, place eight to ten drops of your desired oil into the water and relax for twenty minutes. I suggest *Calming Essential Oil Blend* (which features lavender) to relax, *Energize Essential Oil Blend* to revive, and *Muscle Soothe Essential Oil Blend* for use after sports or for tired, sore muscles.
- For colds and flu, use three drops of lavender and three drops of tea tree oil.
- For children, I suggest five to seven drops of lavender essential oil or *Calming* blend to calm, kill germs, and boost the immune system.
- For babies (newborn to two years old), use three to five drops of lavender or *Calming* blend.

COMPRESS

- Add ten drops of essential oil or essential oil blend to a bowl of water. Place a cloth into the water, remove, and ring it out, then place it onto the affected area. This method is best for large rashes, chicken pox, poison ivy, and poison oak. For children, use lavender or *Calming* oil blend. For adults, combine *Calming* or lavender oil and two to three drops of peppermint.

MASSAGE

- If you visit a massage therapist, request that your favorite essential oil be added to her/his carrier oil. Lots of essential oils are good for massage. Or bring along *Earth Tribe Massage Oil* or *Body Oil* for the massage therapist.
- If you don't see a massage therapist regularly, figure out a way to start! Alternatively, you could take a partners massage class with someone special or learn self-massage techniques. Or do all three. You will be healthier, happier, and much less stressed for it.

sore throats. Herbalists offer recipes combining lavender, lemon, eucalyptus, and rosemary oils to quiet chest colds and coughs.

It is important to realize that not all lavender oils are equally therapeutic. Too many products have been wrongly processed and have stripped away the plant's effectiveness. Or less potent species of lavender are used to save money for the manufacturers.

Lavendula angustifolia plants are what aromatherapists call "true lavender." Essential oil of this lavender originally grown in high altitude is rare, but reputable companies do offer highly effective lavender essential oils.

True lavender is a remarkable painkiller and healing agent for wounds and burns. It is worth the expense if you can find it.

Just make sure there's actually essential oil in those soaps. Or better yet, use the essential oils yourself. It's a small step, but one with big potential.

Chapter 2

Essential Oils 101: The Short Course

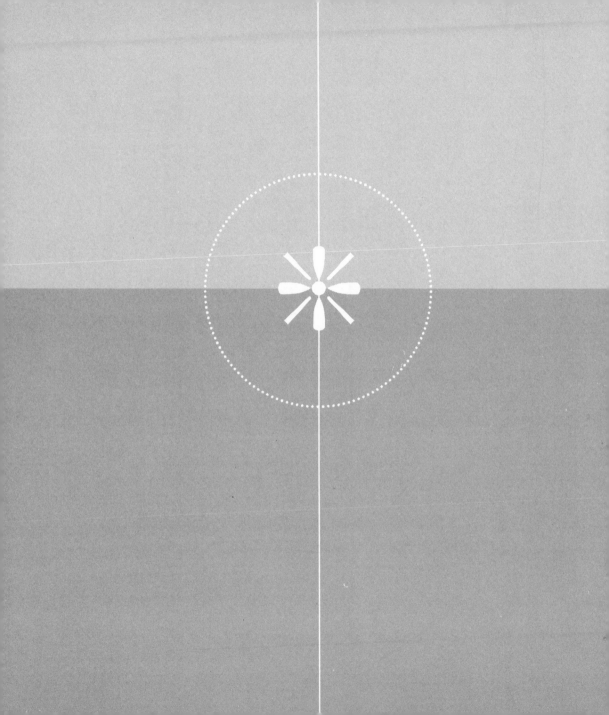

Forget everything you know or

have heard about aromatherapy . . . at least for a few moments. Let's start from scratch—and certainly not just sniff.

The term *aromatherapy* is confusing because plant oils don't have to be directly inhaled for healing benefits. Far from it. In fact, researchers are finding humans may have a sixth sense that doesn't use the senses of smell, sight, hearing, touch, or taste but nonetheless detects and absorbs chemicals in the air that can modify our conscious or unconscious behavior.

Scientists have known for decades that fish, reptiles, and a good number of other mammals—apes, dogs, and elephants—transmit and receive silent signals that help them to fall in love, reproduce, maintain social status, define territories, and express and dictate moods. Now they are finding that humans experience a similar activity through a tiny structure in the nose called the vomeronasal organ (VNO).

There is still a lot of debate about exactly how and if the VNO consistently sends signals to the brain—whether it is to relax, feel more confident, or gauge attraction to others—but a growing number of mainstream scientists are investigating the possibilities. For instance, researchers at the University of Chicago's highly respected Institute for Mind and Biology have published several major papers on the VNO during the last few years, while prominent European psychologists are convinced this sixth sense will predict success in love, work, and life.

This is big stuff. I repeat, this is big stuff. Twenty years from now, we will wonder what took so long to scent homes or workplaces with essential oils or why American doctors didn't use plant oils as remedies sooner. We will better understand that essential oils can help free our environment and Earth of toxins—and might provide our best chance to reverse disturbing trends, and make a natural difference with the little things in life, too.

The heightened interest of the scientific community is a sure sign that essential oils of plants are going to become integral to maintaining everyday health and well-being in the decades ahead. Consider my Healthy Living plan as your head start to being on the cutting edge.

None of these new findings diminishes the value of inhaling plant oils or what is commonly known as aromatherapy, quite the contrary. Unlike the senses of sight, touch, hearing, and taste—which travel via the central nervous system to the brain's thalamus, which in turn evaluates the sensations and only then delivers messages to the cortex of the brain for appropriate action—nerve signals created from smell go directly to the brain's limbic system. This region of the brain controls our moods and emotions, which explains why fresh-cut grass, just-baked pie, or a bouquet of flowers can immediately transport us to another time and place in our minds. Our sense of smell sends signals for appetite, digestion, sexual arousal, memory, body temperature, and heartbeat directly to the brain, bypassing the central nervous system.

The limbic system is also instrumental in regulating heart rate and muscle tension among other functions. The proper scent—peppermint oil for example—can send limbic signals to enhance mental alertness. Vanilla has been used to calm patients undergoing lengthy MRI procedures.

As some natural health physicians have speculated, using inhalation therapy seems far too simplistic for mainstream doctors, yet in reality the whole process is probably too complex, and intricately effective, for us to completely understand its potential.

I want to make a similar point about the body absorbing plant oils through the skin, since rubbing plant oils into the skin by massage is a highly effective way to gain healing benefits. Doctors and scientists are increasingly willing to accept that substances can enter the bloodstream through the skin (reversing a position held from the earlier days of Western medicine, which dictated that the skin wouldn't allow most chemicals to penetrate). They no longer doubt that the skin can be a delivery system for the entire body and mind (I would include the soul, too). If you want simple proof, look at the growing number of skin patches prescribed by American doctors. Nicotine patches are used for smoking cessation, nitroglycerin patches deliver relief from angina pain in the heart and chest, and estrogen patches are used for hormone replacement therapy.

The tiny molecules of plant oils make it easy for them to pass through the skin to the bloodstream. Some compounds in oils pass faster than others. It is common knowledge among practitioners that lighter compounds in lavender show up in the bloodstream in about twenty minutes, while eucalyptus and thyme require up to forty minutes; bergamot and lemon take forty to sixty minutes; and geranium, peppermint, and heavier compounds in lavender are absorbed into the bloodstream somewhere between one and two hours.

Along with massage and direct inhalation, plant oils can be used with steam or saunas, diffused through a room (through special lightbulb rings, diffusers, vaporizers, or even a few drops in a bowl of water), applied by hot or cold compress, or added to a hot bath. Each of these techniques helps the body get the maximum benefits from the oils through the sense of smell, absorption through the skin, or VNO sensation.

Testing, Testing . . .

Nonbelievers can try this test to be persuaded that plant oils can enter the skin and make their way throughout the blood, brain, and other parts of the body. Slice a clove of garlic in half, then rub the cut side on the soles of your feet liberally. Put on a pair of socks. About twenty minutes later, you will have garlic breath. It won't do much for your social prowess, but it demonstrates my point!

So aromatherapy is not a bad word, it's just incomplete. There is more to making yourself the total picture of health and well-being.

That's why I prefer to focus on essential oils of plants as the cornerstone of my Healthy Living plan. The essential oils of plants are derived from seeds, bark, roots, leaves, flowers, wood, balsam, and resin. The oils come from glands deep inside the plant's cells and make plants fragrant. Essential oils give herbs, spices, flowers, and fruit their specific scent or flavor.

Plants vary in how much essential oil they contain. Lemon is bursting with oil in the glandular cells of its outer peel, while it can require 4,500 to 5,000 pounds of rose petals to produce sixteen ounces. In contrast, it takes about 200 to 250 pounds of lavender plants to make sixteen ounces of lavender oil. What's more, the same plant can yield different oils, such as orange oil from orange peel and neroli oil from orange blossoms.

Essential oils contain hundreds of compounds, many of which haven't been identified yet. You can draw a comparison to the various "phytochemicals" available in vegetables, fruits, grains, seeds, and nuts; researchers admit they don't even know close to half of the healthful compounds in plant foods. What everyone agrees on is that plants are powerful healers and that we have lost our way in using them to aid in wellness and illness. I can help you change that in your life, one step at a time.

Cultivation methods, climate, location, precise botanical species, extraction techniques, and handling have all been found to have a profound effect on the final makeup of an oil. This affects fragrance, purity, and therapeutic value. We will discuss identifying the best oils in the next chapter.

Spirit Break

Many centuries ago, alchemists recognized the inner purity and healing power of plant oils, labeling them "essential." Back then, since fragrance has always been invisible, people considered plant oils to be magical and difficult to define or capture. The comparison was made between trying to describe the power of the oils and the essence of a person's soul: easy to define, no; essential to one's nature, yes.

Not surprisingly, essential oils have been incorporated into ancient spiritual ceremonies by everyone from Hindus to Catholics to Buddhists, and are still widely used today. They are also popular in Native American, African, and Japanese Shinto practices.

For now, I will say this: Be sure any essential oil you plan to try is the real thing. I was in a store the other day and was flabbergasted to see a lavender soap from a big company that didn't contain a single drop of pure lavender. It's important that people maintain a critical eye and be discriminating when buying aromatherapy products. Low-quality oils or the use of solvents or chemicals in the distillation process destroys the therapeutic value and alters the fragrance. The distillation of essential oils is a delicate and precise process.

In the last couple of centuries, with the advancement of scientific principles, essential oils have gained another name, *volatile oils*, because these plant oils are relatively thin (compared to, say, vegetable oils for

Respect the Power of Pure Plant Oils

The potency of pure essential oils is an important matter. Remember, these plant oils are highly concentrated. You need only a few drops for inhalation, diffusion, compresses, and the like. Be sure not to overdo it or fall into the faulty thinking that if a little is good, more is better. Don't follow the lead of manufacturers of household cleaners, who make products entirely too strong for the task.

If you intend to use plant oils for massage, be sure to use the recommended number of drops in a carrier oil such as almond, avocado, grapeseed, soybean, apricot kernel, olive, hazelnut, or canola. Generally speaking, you should never apply most essential oils directly to the skin without a carrier oil (an approximate proportion is four to six drops of essential oil to two tablespoons of carrier oil); do so only if a qualified practitioner directs it. **And never take plant oils internally. They are medicinal and can be toxic when used incorrectly.** Remember that essential oils can indeed detoxify your body, and that detoxification can sometimes lead to minor rashes, headaches, and nausea.

Of course, when you use them wisely, plant oils can replace many of the medicines and over-the-counter synthetic remedies in your bathroom cabinet, along with overhauling the supplies under your kitchen sink. You will be honoring nature's powerful healing agents and stemming the tide of artificial chemicals in our world. That's a win-win situation of the best kind.

cooking), usually don't leave oily stains on cloth, and evaporate quickly into the air. Volatile means "vaporous" or to be "like gas."

But that doesn't mean the healing effect of plant oil is fleeting. The oil's molecules are tiny enough to penetrate the skin and reach the most hard-to-navigate portions of nasal and brain passages. They prompt many positive responses in the body, such as signaling the brain to relax muscles or sharpening attention. Scientists believe essential oils remain in the body for maybe three or four hours at most, which is a significant advantage in avoiding the side effects of drugs that remain in the body for days or even weeks. Even with the short stay, essential oils may trigger healing responses that can continue for days or possibly weeks.

For a hint at what essential oils can do for the body and soul, understand that they protect plants against disease and play a vital role in the life cycle of plants. Essential oils are literally essential to the survival of plants. Some researchers liken them to hormones in the human body, which are increasingly regarded as the primary factor to maintaining health or falling ill, especially in the case of women.

In fact, a recent study showed that men who lose certain hormones at a faster rate in middle age than other males will suffer disrupted deep-sleep patterns. You will learn in Chapter 4 how essential oils can help fight insomnia and promote better rest at night.

Medicine Cabinet

Herbalists and aromatherapists know that what essential oils do for plants they can perform for humans, too. Here are some of the medicinal properties of plant oils:

- Protect the body and kill harmful bacteria, viruses, and funguses
- Reduce inflammation
- Regulate hormone levels in the body
- Tend wounds and cuts faster and without scarring
- Stimulate the immune system
- Tone and moisturize skin
- Treat skin conditions such as rosacea and eczema
- Repel insects (although some flower fragrances do serve as nature's call to bees)
- Aid in digestion
- Increase oxygen intake and availability to individual cells
- Decrease sinus and respiratory congestion
- Balance emotions and reduce anxiety

Take Note

At *Earth Tribe*, we refer to our primary line of essential oils as *single notes*. They are the pure thing. Here's a look at our most popular oils and what they can do for you and your family:

- Bergamot: Cheerful and uplifting, often used in European clinics to treat depression. Also used for anxiety/stress relief, for mind–body balance, to curb mood swings, and as an immune system booster. Part of the citrus fruit family.
- Eucalyptus: Cools the body in summer and protects it in winter. Used as a disinfectant, an insect repellant, and a decon-

gestant; for relief from sinus pain and sore muscles; to reduce acne/blemishes; and to promote mind–body balance.

• Geranium: Wonderful worn alone as a perfume and extremely uplifting. Works well for female energy. Also good for anxiety/stress relief, depression, menopause symptoms, and PMS. In addition it normalizes dry or oily skin and promotes hormonal balance.

• Grapefruit: Terrific oil for the kitchen, helps eliminate odors and cuts grease. Acts as an astringent and facial toner. Also used for cellulite, lymphatic drainage, and water retention.

• Juniper: Highly rejuvenating in the bath. Helps reduce water retention. Acts as an astringent and toxin eliminator. Energizing and invigorating.

• Lavender: The most gentle and versatile oil as we learned in Chapter 1. Excellent for children/infants' baths. Highly calming. Also used to treat blemishes, burns, insomnia, nervous tension, rashes, scrapes/cuts, and sunburn.

• Lemon: Carries solar vitality to the body, mind, and soul. Think of it as the sun's golden gift. Refreshes and revives, disinfects, but remember to never use directly on skin without diluting with carrier oil such as avocado, grapeseed, or sweet almond oil. Used for stress relief, depression, cold and flu symptoms, and cleaning.

• Orange: Great scent for kids. Ideal in the kitchen as a freshener. Can be an effective insect repellant. Used for depression, lymphatic drainage, and to decrease wrinkles.

- Patchouli: Basic ingredient of many classic erogenous perfumes. Works as an aphrodisiac. Helps you feel grounded. Also used to balance emotions, soothe dry skin, and repel insects.
- Peppermint: Cooling after a workout or other strenuous activity. Use with base oil as an after-workout spray or add some drops to your bath or shower. Also used to help with muscle pain, digestive problems, bad breath, and headaches.
- Rose: The symbol for love, sensuality, and compassion. Helps release anger and grief. Works as an antiseptic and infection fighter. Used to help with PMS discomfort and insomnia, to encourage cell rejuvenation, and to heal eczema and broken capillaries.
- Rosemary: Protective scent that helps clear negative energy from one's aura and environment. Energizing. Effective in treating headaches, promoting mental concentration, and enhancing memory.
- Sandalwood: Woodsy, earthy scent offers meditative qualities. Can be used as an aphrodisiac and sexual restorative for men and women, and also as an appetite depressant, a sedative, and a stress reliever.
- Tea tree: Currently one of the most studied essential oils because it can help treat both bacterial and viral infections, plus athlete's foot, acne, cold sores, gum problems, flu symptoms, insect bites, rashes, and yeast infections.

History

I have always felt a little bit that René-Maurice Gattefosse and I are soul mates of sorts. He was the French chemist who in 1928 discovered the healing benefits of lavender oil by accident. He was working in the lab of his family's perfume business when he severely burned his hands. He reached for the closest substance to soothe the burn, which happened to be a beaker of lavender oil. What he discovered was that the lavender not only eased his immediate pain but also sped his healing process.

Gattefosse pursued his study of essential oils of plants and published his research on the subject. He referred to his discovery as aromatherapy because the lavender smelled so good, even though, oddly enough, he never delved much into how oils worked when they were inhaled.

That part of the essential oil equation fell to another Frenchman, Dr. Jean Valnet. He was a pioneer in using essential oils for specific physical and mental conditions, and his 1964 book on the subject has been widely translated (in English as *The Practice of Aromatherapy*) and has inspired countless physicians and health practitioners in Europe. Among his most important discoveries was the fact that essential oils can kill bacteria, viruses, and funguses when sprayed into the air. While serving as a surgeon in the army during World War II, he used essential oils as an antiseptic. He identified essential oils as especially valuable as antiseptics because of their aggression toward microbial germs and safety for healthy tissue.

We are just starting to catch up to the concept in this country. I say essential oils are the most important rediscovery of our times, and will only become more so in the decades ahead as we struggle with bacteria that are becoming resistant to antibiotic drugs.

Aromatherapy may sound like a New Age development to skeptics, but it is actually one of the oldest industries in the world. The earliest study of aromatherapy most likely began when humans first learned to use fire. By throwing different branches or twigs on the fire, they would have noticed how certain burning plants changed the demeanor of those near the fire, and how others kept insects away. Over time, humans discovered that the fragrant substance, its essential oil, could be pressed from the plant and used in a variety of ways.

Diffusing the Situation

One of the simplest ways to disperse essential oils in a room is to use a clay pot diffuser. As an added bonus, these convenient devices are inexpensive.

Clay pot diffusers can be found in various small shapes such as pyramids. The typical diffuser has an opening for adding essential oils that is closed by a cork. By design, the oils permeate through the terra-cotta pot (which is glazed on the bottom) and then slowly diffuse out into the room. The intensity of the aroma depends on how much essential oil is added to the clay pot.

Along with ease of use and inexpensiveness, what I like best about clay pot diffusers is that the oil is not heated and consequently altered in any way.

The documented roots of essential oils and aromatherapy go back to about 400 B.C. The ancient Chinese used plant oils as medicines, while ancient Egyptian high priests employed them for preparing the dead for afterlife and other religious ceremonies. It is said that Cleopatra was a masterful aromatherapist, using plant essences to scent herself and the palace to seduce her men. Her daily baths featured rose oil, one of the most precious of all oils to this day. She even scented the sails of her ship when departing to meet Mark Antony, inspiring the famous Shakespeare passage, "The winds were lovesick."

References to essential oils appear in the Bible more than 150 times, one being the mention that the Three Wise Men brought myrrh and frankincense among their gifts. The famed Greek physician Hippocrates— the one who wrote the oath our doctors still swear to—urged the burning of aromatic plants in the streets to protect Greeks from the plague. He wrote, "The way to health is to have an aromatic bath and a scented massage every day." Now, no offense to apple growers, but that's my kind of prescription for wellness!

For maximum therapeutic effect, it is necessary to use a forced-air, no-heat diffuser, such as *Earth Tribe's Nebulizing Diffuser.* It is the next step up from a clay pot diffuser, if you are willing to make the investment. Here is a list of frequently asked questions from the *Earth Tribe* Internet site (www.earth-tribe.com) about nebulizing diffusers:

1. How does a nebulizer work?

Essential oils are vaporized, or atomized in the lower chamber by pressure from the air pump. Before the atomized essential oil(s) can exit the nebulizer, it travels over several glass baffles that allow the finer droplets (between one and four microns) to be released into the air.

You benefit from this action in two ways: (1) Droplets of this size stay suspended in the air for long periods of time, maximizing the benefits; and (2) when inhaled, these tiny droplets are considered the optimum size for deep therapeutic action.

The glass baffles act as vortex generators and create a substantial amount of turbulence, which ionizes the essential oil vapor as it leaves the nebulizer. Many researchers believe this ionic charge on the oil molecules is an important and integral part of the therapeutic process. For example, Charlene Eastman at the University of Illinois–Chicago sleep disorders center has found negative ion generators can help relieve symptoms of seasonal affective disorder (SAD), also known as winter depression.

2. Where do I put the essential oil?

The essential oil sits in the bowl part of the glass fixture. To fill the bowl, you simply take the directional tip off and drop oil through the top. Unlike other models, the *Earth Tribe* model has no metal or plastic parts that come into contact with the essential oil. If essential oil comes into contact with metal, it can change the chemical composition of the oil, and if it comes into contact with plastic over a long period of time, the plastic breaks down.

3. Can I use anything else in a nebulizing diffuser?

No, you should use only natural essential oils, not fragrance oils. Diffusing fragrance oils into the air is unhealthy, and fragrance oils may clog

Simone Stahl

Fifteen months old was a scary time for Max Stahl and his mother, Simone. Max was deathly ill. The doctors kept telling Simone the condition was caused by a virus, and that they expected it to clear up.

Little Max was always sick with upper respiratory infections, coughing, and wheezing. By the time Max was eighteen months, Simone says, "we knew something was not right." Max no longer had the energy to lift his head off the pillow. He had no energy to play or eat. He quit talking.

Worse, Max was down to one, maybe two bottles of milk a day. Simone and her husband, Duane, were fed up. They figured the viral diagnosis was more a way for doctors to put a label on the condition rather than do something about curing it.

"I wanted something done before we were going to lose Max," Simone recalls. "He was pale with dark circles under his eyes. The whites of his eyes were gray. He was the picture of death."

The Stahls took Max yet again to the pediatrician, who sent them to see a gastroenterologist the next day. The specialist took one look at Max and said, "We have a very sick little boy."

Simone sobbed right there in the medical office. Max was worked up for brain tumors and leukemia and had a GI tube placed. He was to be tube-fed for eight weeks. His lab results were inconclusive. The MRI, CAT scan, and ultrasounds were negative.

Several specialists—hematologist, dietitian, occupational therapist, physical therapist, lung specialist—and thousands of dollars later, it was the allergist who diagnosed Max with severe allergies. Simone had kept her dear friend Mooney informed about Max's progress—or lack of it. Leslie suggested that the Stahls get rid of their usual household cleaning products and try a more natural approach to housework. Leslie told Simone about essential oils, and how they naturally purify the air without the toxic odors and residues.

Simone decided to give it a try. As a registered nurse, she had exhausted the medical system and sought the advice of the best experts she could find. Leslie sent some *Earth Tribe* oils, and Max's symptoms improved tenfold in just a few weeks.

Max was ill from May 1998 until September 1999. Simone started using the essential oils for household cleaning that September and Max has been clear of illness ever since. He is off his nebulizer treatments, off inhalers, finally gaining weight, and no longer has a chronic runny nose. Max is as healthy as the typical four-year-old.

"If anyone suffers allergies I would rethink what toxic waste is in the home and what can be done to improve the quality of the home environment," says Simone, who is now an *Earth Tribe* sales consultant. "Essential oils have been a godsend for us, and they might do just the same for the health of your family."

the nebulizer. Also, thick resins or oils like patchouli and sandalwood should be blended with thinner oils before diffusing.

4. How do I clean the nebulizer?

Remove the nebulizer glass from the pump, pour out any unused oil, and rinse the glass with rubbing alcohol or hydrogen peroxide. It is best not to let any unused oil sit in the glass nebulizer for more than a few days, as it will thicken and clog the diffuser. If that should occur, gooey oil and clogs can be easily removed by soaking the glass nebulizer in rubbing alcohol.

5. How long should I run the oil?

As long as you want; nothing bad will happen, even if you run out of oil. The pump is designed to run twenty-four hours a day, seven days a week. But to deliver a proper aromatherapy treatment, you really do not need to run the diffuser more than thirty to forty-five minutes. That is enough to saturate the air with the healing effects of the oils. For convenience, you can plug the diffuser into an ordinary household lamp timer.

Chapter 3

The PLANT
Lifestyle

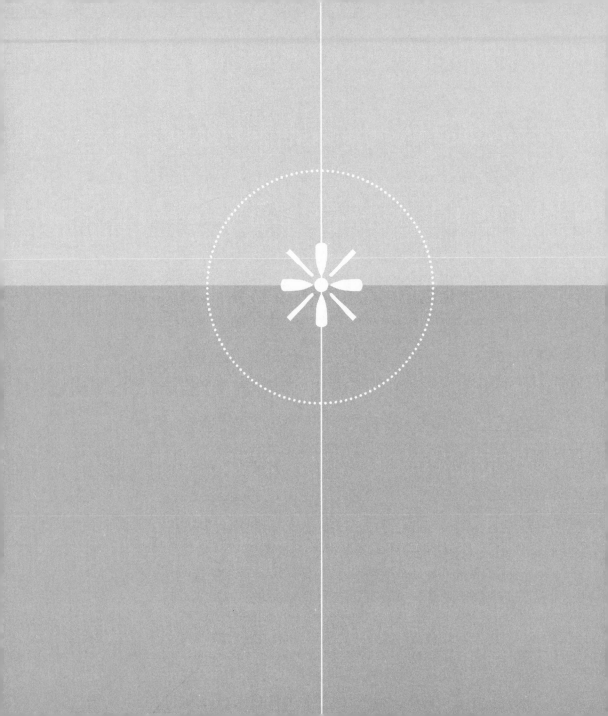

This is a chapter about questions. Mostly ones you need to ask yourself about how essential oils and my Healthy Living plan can fit into your life—rather than you fitting into the plan. Plant oils can fit into anyone's lifestyle or busy schedule. There is no extensive time commitment and the oils are easy to use. That's why I think of my plan as being for "everyone, every day."

You might say everyone has a *healthstyle*. Researchers and health practitioners will all advise us on the best foods to eat or exercises to do, but the strategies don't work unless people follow them. Each of us decides, by our actions, what it is we are willing to do for personal health. We might talk about change or aspire to it, but doing something about it is usually another story.

It is so easy to use plant oils to help you remake your lifestyle that you will hardly know you're doing anything differently. You do it by taking small, doable steps. Many of the top researchers who study behavioral change now realize that getting people to move in a positive direction in increments, not one swooping change, is the key to success and an improved healthstyle.

I have developed a convenient checklist of questions you can use to evaluate whether an essential oil works with your healthstyle. You can remember it in the form of an acronym, PLANT, which stands for questions about Purpose, Length of time, Accessibility, Natural ingredients, and Teaching. Let's take a look at each category:

Question Session

Ask yourself these five basic questions before deciding if any essential oil or related product fits into your healthstyle:

1. What is my **Purpose** for using the oil?

2. What is the **Length of time** it will take to show results?

3. Is the oil **Accessible** in my life?

4. Is the oil or product **Natural**?

5. Am I **Teaching** others how to use the oils?

Purpose

Asking yourself why you have decided to use an essential oil—or to eat better, work out more, or meditate—might seem too obvious. We all know eating right or exercising regularly can improve personal health. Meditating or filling a diffuser with essential oils at bedtime will naturally enhance our peace of mind. But there is a significant gap between knowing something is good for us and embracing it as a consistent act in our everyday lives.

What closes the gap is finding a deeper purpose in the new health habit. I don't want you to use essential oils because I endorse them or run a company that makes and sells them. My goal is to help you discover how plant oils can make you feel better physically, emotionally, mentally, and spiritually each and every day. I want people to connect the dots in their own lives, using the best oils for them to create a picture of whole health. It's about you, not me.

The better personal trainers and nutritionists understand this point. They know their ultimate success with any client is getting the individual to become self-motivated. Those newly inspired runners or breakfast eaters have discovered a lasting reason to follow their routines. It might make them feel more energetic. Self-esteem strengthens along with muscle tissue. Mental alertness can improve. They eventually run or eat better for themselves, not because a trainer or nutritionist is checking up on them. In fact, the top trainers and nutritionists realize that if they do their jobs well enough, some clients won't need them anymore. All of which is okay because those happy clients are referring friends and loved ones left and right.

Without purpose, we slip back into unhealthy patterns sooner or later. A wedding or reunion might be motivation enough for losing weight, but the pounds stay off only when people see how they are less tired at the end of the day or feel more hopeful about the future. They feel lighter in ways beyond the bathroom scale.

You may have specific health reasons for trying the plant oils outlined in my plan. Or your goal might be to increase energy and reduce stress, which is a winning change in life's equation for any of us. Whatever your goal, the purpose runs deeper.

With the first decision to use an oil or two, you may be getting started on the strength of a goal. That's perfectly okay. Goals are good kick-starts. But what you should try to do is to seek out the deeper purpose. You might be using rosemary oil for headaches and then find it is actually increasing your mental concentration and allowing you to learn more about the people and things around you. You feel more engaged with the world—and not a single aspirin is necessary.

Plant oils work on symptoms, but more important, they help you reconnect to yourself. I think plant oils can help us resurrect the art form of healing and add more meaning to our lives. The essence of plants—the most precious and embedded cells of nature—will work wonders for the body and mind. Even better, they open up the path to self-discovery.

So before using any oil, be sure to understand why you are planning to use it. Asking the question up front will help you recognize the answer when it begins to appear in your life. The process might start with a goal, but always look for the underlying purpose (which gets easier as you begin using more than one oil). Your life will be stronger and more vibrant for it.

Length of Time

The next question in my PLANT approach is: What is the length of time it takes for essential oils to work?

There is no one answer here. For improving mood or relieving stress, it might be a New York minute—literally. When Duke University researchers sprayed pleasant food aromas (such as baked apple pie) in subway cars, they found there was 40 percent less pushing and shoving during crowded rush-hour rides and fewer nasty comments per minute. At Memorial Sloan-Kettering Cancer Center in Manhattan, patients who inhaled vanilla-scented air while undergoing magnetic resonance imaging (MRI) screening experienced significantly less anxiety than a control group. If those same researchers used essential oils—say juniper or geranium for subway cars and lavender for MRIs—the results would be even better because the oils are many times more potent.

If you are using essential oils to clear up a medical condition, it might take days or weeks to notice results. In any case, it is a good idea to talk to your health practitioner about your plan to use plant oils, not so much to get approval as to make sure you are not forgoing treatment that can speed your healing. Where plant oils work so effectively is in healing the body—and mind and soul—rather than simply masking symptoms, which is the effect of too many drugs on the market. But that healing

"No Time at All"

There is another question about plant oils and length of time: How long do they take to use each day? The answer is a happy one: practically no time at all! You can basically add essential oils to your day in a matter of seconds or, at most, a few minutes. That's why my Healthy Living program works for everyone, every day. Plus, essential oils themselves can have an initial effect on the human body within ten seconds!

might require more time than we are accustomed to in today's quick-fix society.

Another positive aspect of involving your health practitioner, or another qualified person such as a personal coach or nutritionist, is to help you gauge your progress. They can provide trained feedback at regular intervals. Keeping a brief journal of your daily condition is another good idea (try physical, emotional, mental, and spiritual categories or heart, mind, and soul if you prefer). I recommend that clients keep it short. For instance, promise yourself to write for no more than a minute.

Boosting energy is a common goal for all of us. You will likely feel different from the first drops, though the real payoff unfolds in the days and weeks ahead. Using plant oils to feel stronger and more grounded is a longer process than, say, drinking a triple espresso, but the positive effects will last a lot longer!

Accessibility

An important factor about any essential oil is accessibility. Does it fit into your daily routine?

Most of us are foiled in our health plans more by ambition than laziness. We decide to make too many changes too fast. With plant oils, I always recommend starting with one product, making it part of your life before moving on to other ideas. So pick what's bothering you most—headaches, using too many chemicals around the home, relationship tumult—and look for an oil to help you address it. You will feel more in control of the situation, and you'll give yourself the chance to determine if the oil is helping you or not.

It may be that you receive an essential oil kit as a gift, or you purchase a starter kit like we sell at *Earth Tribe*. That's a great concept, just don't try to use everything at once. Introduce new oils on a weekly or bi-weekly basis, depending on your own schedule.

Part of the accessibility factor is whether you can easily acquire the product. This is an increasingly easier proposition. While lots of stores sell what they call aromatherapy and plant oil products, chances are most of those offerings are not pure enough to be therapeutic. But once you find a reliable company, you will likely be able to order by phone or computer without much trouble.

Money can be an accessibility issue, since the best-made plant oils are costly to produce. But don't be swayed by significantly less expensive versions of plant oils. They will undoubtedly be ripoffs and truly a waste of your money. With pure oils, mere drops can make a flood of difference.

Natural Products

Is the oil natural? This is a key question and an important link in my PLANT approach to using essential oils.

Your primary concern in purchasing any essential oil or blend of oils should be to make sure there are no synthetic ingredients. In fact, some oils are synthetic altogether. It shouldn't surprise you to discover that today scientists can closely re-create practically any aroma in the laboratory with chemicals. But that synthetic oil—or oils with synthetic main ingredients used to stretch the more costly plant oil—just won't produce the same effect on the brain and body compared to a pure plant oil. The molecular structure is different. Another problem with synthetic oils or fragrances is that they come with a greater risk of allergic reactions, such as skin rashes, sneezing, headaches, and puffy eyes. In fact, the U.S. Environmental Protection Agency classifies synthetic fragrances in the same category as pesticides and heavy metal solvents for potential adverse health effects.

Once you learn how pure essential oils smell, you will be able to distinguish between the real thing and the fake. It won't take long before you realize there are a lot of impostors out there.

Sometimes it is easy enough to spot synthetic oils, like when a store sells, say, peach, strawberry, or lilac oil on the same brand display with "essential" oils. None of those three can be produced readily naturally—they have to be made synthetically. It's likely the rest of the line is synthetic, too.

Similarly, you might see vanilla, jasmine, or rose oil selling much lower than the typical $60 to $70 per one-eighth ounce (which is obviously on the way-high side for essential oils but can be worth the price if the oil solves a major problem, such as a chronic skin condition). That's a tipoff the oils are synthetic or use artificial ingredients in much greater proportion to the essential plant oil.

More Tips

Check out the labels. Manufacturers are supposed to list ingredients in order of largest amount to smallest. If there are any synthetic ingredients, keep looking. You want pure oils. If the label does not list ingredients, that's a sure sign you might not be getting what you pay for, or, more important, what your body needs.

Earth Healing
Charlotte Rich

Charlotte Rich is a Los Angeles–based singer who can't afford any unnecessary drains on her health in the competitive entertainment business. For years, though, she battled recurring cold sores that always seemed to pop up at the most inopportune times—before a big audition or opening night. She visited a doctor for the cold sores, but his prescription creams and ointments never really seemed to help much. Then she discovered tea tree oil and the world seemed a less draining place.

"I would suffer with the cold sores after each outbreak for about ten days," says Charlotte. "These days I use *Earth Tribe Tea Tree Oil,* which has natural antiviral properties. Now if I feel a sore coming on, I apply it topically to relieve the throbbing and contain the outbreak."

Some essential oils are diluted on purpose by producers to make them more affordable or to offer them in a convenient form, such as the *Earth Tribe Claire* spray, which is terrific for freshening stale air. Some people don't want to make their own blends, household cleaners, or beauty products (you will learn how with "recipes" throughout this book). *Earth Tribe* and other reputable manufacturers can do it for you at reasonable prices.

Remember, there is nothing wrong with diluting essential oils with pure carrier oils, including jojoba, almond, or grapeseed. You almost always need to dilute them before use. Once you become more familiar with the various oils, you might want to make your own recipes for some jobs and buy the more convenient products for others. Pick whatever best fits your lifestyle.

"Warning Signs"

Watch out for these synthetic oils. They can't match pure essential oils for healing and energizing the body:

Apple

Coconut

Gardenia

Lilac

Magnolia

New-mown hay

Peach

Rain

Raspberry

Strawberry

Lesson Plan

You can get creative while being proactive about teaching others in your life about the healing and energizing power of plant oils. You can put together a starter kit gift to get the discussion off on the right foot. Other ideas? Well, ahem, you can buy someone special a copy of this book. Plus, look for a product that would fit into that person's lifestyle. At *Earth Tribe*, we sell *Owie Juice* that kids love to spray on cuts and scrapes. Guys love our *Muscle Soothe* formula featuring sweet birch and peppermint oils to relieve sore or overworked muscles and joints. Someone with sleep troubles would appreciate our *Sweet Dreams* blend (with the main ingredients of marjoram and lavender) to improve rest. And the frequent traveler in your life (maybe that's you!) will soon go nowhere without our *Tummy Tonic*, which features peppermint and ginger essential oils for the stress and upset stomachs that can come with spending too much time in airports and airplanes.

Teaching

Are you making sure to teach the right people in your life how to use essential oils? Simply introducing a plant oil such as lavender to your household might not be enough. Start by teaching yourself how to use it for calming, but don't stop there. Demonstrate the technique—in this case we are talking about misting a child's room at night or putting a few drops on your own pillow—to your spouse or kids or baby-sitter. They can become converts, too, and their cooperation will save you time and worry.

Informing others about plant oils and how to use them takes some pressure off of you and makes the world a healthier place! Who knows—your spouse or kids or other loved ones (don't forget friends and co-workers) might become even more fascinated with essential oils than you, and they may even teach you some valuable lessons in the process.

Chapter 4

The Body's Wake-up Call

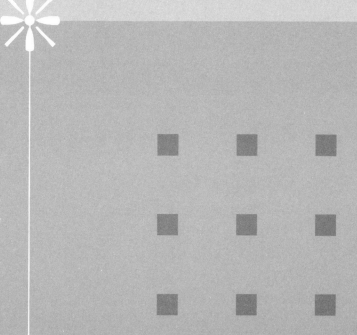

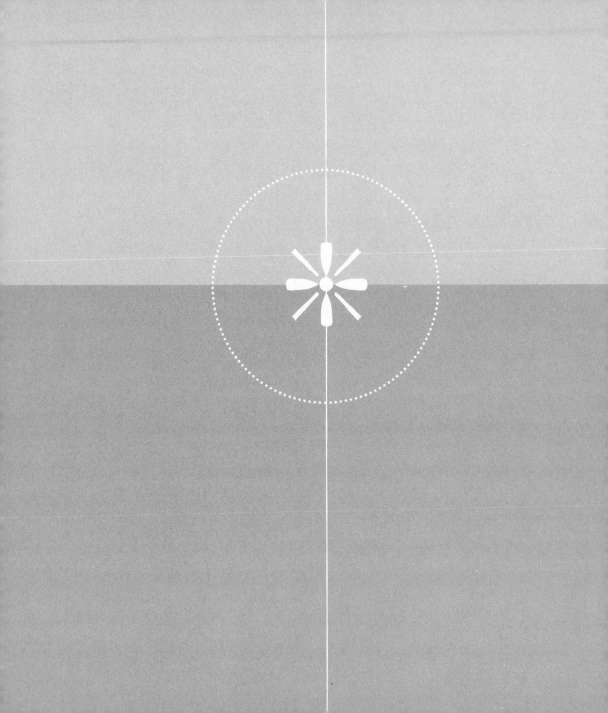

Let's talk about what I consider the greatest, truly natural resource we all possess: *personal energy*. The trouble is, it is too frequently in short supply. Life and its stresses have a way of tapping our energy.

Now, I agree that physical activity, which requires some energy output but pays off by giving more back, is a terrific way to feel better. I make yoga part of my days and weeks for the physical, emotional, mental, and spiritual energy it can provide me. Eating healthy foods is another valuable strategy. I say stay as close as possible to whole plant foods for nature's powerhouse of nutrients. Load up on the fruits, vegetables, whole grains, nuts, and seeds.

Think about wellness as one of those pie charts. Each of us has a different equation. One slice might be running, another slice could be a yoga practice. An admirable slice is to eat plenty of fruits and vegetables. My biggest slice, day in and day out, is the use of essential oils and the elimination of synthetic chemicals in my life and my husband's and children's lives.

Essential oils are your single best source for boosting your current energy level. It can help every one of us, every day. And not unimportant, using plant oils takes less time than exercise or nutrition. It's even faster than brewing a cup of coffee!

Using essential oils is a twofold benefit. You get the benefit of the oils and avoid synthetic chemicals in a world that, let's face it, is already way too harsh. Here's how the one-two combination works:

- Plant oils can relieve stress and anxiety, help regulate mood and emotions, act as a natural antidepressant, stimulate focus and memory, encourage meditation, and set ideal conditions for romance and relationships.
- We live in a world that accepts twenty-two synthetic ingredients in a leading brand-name soap. We can subtract countless chemicals from our daily lives by using essential oils as the active ingredients in our soaps, shampoos, skin toners, moisturizers, perfumes, and other personal care and beauty items.

And that's just a start! I will show you how to detoxify every room in your home or office and even positively influence the people around you, including your lover.

There is *addition by subtraction* for your healthstyle in simply eliminating chemicals and other harsh additives from your life. Adding essential oils just makes life even better—and more natural.

Strangely enough, one place to look for examples is in the Japanese workforce. For decades, corporate managers in Japan have contracted to have different scents pumped through heating and air-conditioning systems to increase worker productivity and mental concentration. The typical office or factory worker might be treated to lemon oil aromatherapy in the morning to fully awaken them, though alarm clocks that spray stimulating fragrances with the morning buzzer are common. At lunchtime, workers might be inhaling rose oil to unwind, then lemon or peppermint oil in the midafternoon to fight the blahs (circadian rhythm

The Rundown to Avoid Becoming Rundown

Juniper, peppermint, rosemary, and eucalyptus oils each have significant ability to rejuvenate the body. Rosemary addresses the cardiovascular and muscular systems. Sweet birch and peppermint are good for relieving joint aches and pains. Peppermint, highly regarded for settling the digestive tract, is equally effective for clearing the respiratory system and combating headaches. Eucalyptus is good for reducing muscle stiffness.

Moreover, essential oils can be safely used as overall energizers (peppermint, rosemary) or antidepressants (rose, orange, bergamot). Some extracts encourage deeper meditation and relaxation (sandalwood, vetiver, cedarwood, frankincense, myrrh), and some varieties act as aphrodisiacs (clove, ylang ylang, rose).

research shows that most people hit their energy low about four P.M., no matter where they live).

Peppermint oil might be worth more than any number of triple espresso drinks you can imagine. I know clients who use it every afternoon when they get just bored or stressed enough to start thinking about having more coffee or caffeinated sodas as a pick-me-up. Instead, they put a few drops of oil in their diffusers or aromatherapy lightbulb rings. Or they can put the oil in steaming water and inhale.

The same brain waves that are stimulated by caffeine react to the peppermint oil. Only you don't get the rebound effect of coffee or cola, which typically means about thirty minutes later you notice a drop in attention span when caffeine has finished jolting the system. What's happening with coffee is the adrenal glands are pumping extra hormones for the first half-hour—not unlike times when you are panicked or working with an unbending deadline—then the adrenals accommodate the overstimulation by dipping way below normal activity levels.

Caffeine is great while it lasts—maybe even a touch more energizing than plant oils, I admit—but oils keep your brain and adrenal glands at heightened energy levels for hours without any side effects. Just keep inhaling (a good reason to invest in a small diffuser for the office or places you frequent besides home). Essential oils stimulate the adrenal glands, yes, but they also calm the central nervous system. The result for you is a natural and pleasant energy boost without the drop-off.

Studies show the energy boost has its tangible rewards, although feeling more grounded and less frazzled ought to be enough. In one study, researchers found that people who worked forty minutes in a stressful but scented environment identified complicated patterns on a computer screen 88 percent of the time compared to 65 percent accuracy for a control group working under the same conditions but without the scents. Peppermint and cinnamon oils were used. Other research indicates that lemon oils can cut computer errors in half.

Wake Up and Smell the Peppermint

Besides peppermint, try these oils instead of your afternoon coffee, soda, or caffeinated tea. Put them in a diffuser, aromatherapy lightbulb ring, or even a spray bottle with water. If one works best, stick with it. And if you're really hooked on the natural high, you might even substitute your essential oils recipes for a morning caffeine. I said might! This program fits your life, not the other way around. Here are the oils:

Basil
Cinnamon
Ginger
Grapefruit
Jasmine
Juniper
Lemon
Orange
Rosemary

Like any part of life, there are situations in which the sum of the parts is greater than the whole. Just think about the energy and happiness you can feel with your family around you or your best friend, or with a coworker who fits perfectly into the effort behind a big project. Plato's idea, for instance, was that lovers were originally one person. The two parts, separated, strive to become joined again. Similarly there are lots of would-be love affairs between essential plant oils. Sometimes a blend of oils can outstrip any effect of the single note, which might be powerful enough but not quite magical. Consider pumpkin pie, of all things. In scientific studies, men have been overwhelmingly attracted to the scent pumpkin pie. Well, combine cinnamon, clove, and ginger oils, and voilà, you have one happy and attentive guy.

For starters, look to manufacturers to provide you with oil blends that work for you. Then, if your enthusiasm grows strong enough that you

Applying Yourself

As a reminder, here are the application methods for essential oils. Find the one that best fits your life and healthstyle. Or use them all!

- Bath: Add eight to ten drops to water for adults; for children add two to five drops.
- Diffuse: Place a few drops in an aromatherapy lamp, a clay pot, or a humidifier, or use *Earth Tribe Base Spray,* or for maximum health benefits, a nebulizing diffuser.
- Body oil: Add fifty drops to four ounces of unscented carrier oil.
- Face oil: Add ten drops to one ounce of carrier oil.
- Perfume: Wear a drop or two of oil on pulse points.
- Foot massage: Apply directly to the foot, but sparingly. You can focus on reflexology points, such as the sides of the toes for sinus pain.

will commit to making time for it in your busy life, you can move to blending your own oils. *Earth Tribe* makes a full line of blends, but we also offer base sprays and carrier oils to make a starter kit for your own blending.

The process is easy enough but there are some tools of the trade. One is a reducer insert that only allows you to add one drop at a time to your blend (remember, plant oils are highly concentrated). Droppers are another tool, but be careful not to contaminate one oil with another by using the dropper without cleaning it between dips. Convenient-size bottles and containers (for the most part, think small) are usually available at natural foods stores. A notebook (to record successful recipes) and labels (to mark them) are valuable additions to your kitchen laboratory. Be forewarned, once you start blending, it may become habit-forming!

Or you might just prefer blends from my professional essential oils lab to your kitchen, especially if it saves time and fits into your life (do you sense a theme here?). *Earth Tribe* makes an *Energize* blend that combines juniper, peppermint, and geranium. I recommend using it first thing in the morning, before workouts or as an antidote to the afternoon blahs. But the blends don't stop there. Here are other synergistic combinations that are favored by our clients. The names are what we call our products at *Earth Tribe*. Plato would be proud of our matchmaking!

Balance. This blend is the natural solution to the ups and downs of everyday life. Essential oils have been confirmed as effective antidepressants that will balance moods and emotions. Main ingredients: rose, bergamot.

Breathe. A blend of oils carefully formulated to help relieve colds, congestion, sinusitis, and coughs. Main ingredients: eucalyptus, fir.

Calming. A wonderful formulation that helps to melt stress plus induce feelings of tranquility and serenity. Main ingredients: lavender, chamomile.

Courage. Inspired by a Native American tradition in which cedar and pine boughs were rubbed on the body to promote inner strength and purity, and to ground emotions. Pine has been considered *the* cleansing oil for centuries. Main ingredients: spruce, cedarwood.

Detox. This blend is formulated with essential plant oils that aid the body in eliminating toxins and stubborn fatty deposits. Also very helpful for a body that retains water. Main ingredients: juniper, grapefruit, fennel.

Energize. Jump-start your mornings or your workouts, or relieve afternoon energy lows and general fatigue with this stimulating blend. Main ingredients: juniper, peppermint.

Euphoria. A formulation of the oils traditionally known to carry euphoric qualities. Euphoria helps to promote joy, playfulness, and a sense of well-being. Main ingredients: orange, bergamot.

Head Peace. A powerful blend of oils designed to help ease the pain of headaches and migraines, and enhance mental clarity, focus, and vision. Main ingredients: basil, rosemary.

Muscle Soothe. A soothing formulation designed to help alleviate the discomforts of overworked, overstressed muscles, strains and sprains, and sore muscles and joints. Main ingredients: sweet birch, peppermint.

Prosperity. A very special blend of oils that in ancient times were considered more valuable than gold. Based on time-honored tradition, this formula is designed to bring prosperity in health, wealth, family, and love. Main ingredients: frankincense, myrrh.

Sweet Dreams. For restless nights and general insomnia, keep this blend close at hand. A combination of very sedating oils that help to bring on a deep, restful sleep. Main ingredients: marjoram, lavender.

Tummy Tonic. A tummy rub to help alleviate the discomfort of upset stomachs caused by travel, nerves, flu, and over-indulging! Main ingredients: peppermint, ginger.

Another way to visualize the energy in your body is to tap into the Hindu concept of *chakras*. Yoga instructors and energy healers frequently refer to them. In fact, these days, so do some natural health physicians. Chakras are energy centers located at seven points in the body from the base of the spine (known as the first chakra) to the crown of the head (the seventh chakra). An eighth chakra, embraced by some practitioners, would be the radiance or aura that your entire body gives off.

Hindus see the body as an interconnection of energy centers. In the Western world, the idea seems perhaps a bit too metaphysical or far out until you consider that we routinely say things like "He galls me" (which

Some blends are more appropriate for one gender or the other—or when the twain shall meet. Here are some *Earth Tribe* ideas for men, women, and Cupid:

FOR MEN

Recovery. Balancing and stabilizing, this carefully formulated blend supports a balanced connection to earth, aligning body, mind, and spirit. Helps to retain one's unique powers. Balances male energy. Main ingredients: vetiver, cedarwood.

FOR WOMEN

Even Tides. A comforting and balancing formulation specifically designed to help alleviate the uncomfortable symptoms of PMS and menopause. Strengthens and supports female energy. Main ingredients: clary sage, sweet fennel.

Volupte. Earth Tribe's first exotic perfume blend made with 100 percent pure and natural essential oils. As the name implies, this rich blend of rare and precious oils creates a sensuous and pleasurable mood, at the same time promoting a delightfully soothing, warm feeling. Main ingredients: rose, jasmine, frankincense.

FOR ROMANCE

Love. A very romantic blend, formulated with oils that have symbolized and enhanced love throughout time. Makes an enchanting perfume! Main ingredients: ylang ylang, rose.

Night Fire. A provocative combination of nature's aphrodisiacs used for centuries to entice and captivate. This mysterious blend truly sets the mood. Main ingredients: ylang ylang, clove.

can refer to the third chakra in the solar plexus between the navel and rib cage), or "She's a pain the neck" (the fifth chakra, known as the throat chakra, is located in the back of the neck).

Let's investigate each chakra. You might see your own energy imbalances or shortages in between the lines. I have suggested oils you can use to help get back to center, which, believe me, is a place we all want to be. Remember, awareness is always the first step. Knowing about chakras is one baby step, knowing the oils is another. Then pick one chakra and one oil to get started.

- First chakra: Located at the base of the tailbone, it is our foundation. When the first chakra is in sync, we feel grounded.

We accept ourselves. Recommended balancing oils: patchouli, sandalwood, or *Earth Tribe Recovery* blend.

• Second chakra: Located in the lower abdomen, this chakra acts as the primary center for emotions, desires, and the five senses (plus the sixth sense of intuition). It is the hub for creativity and is a good place to target before a big assignment or event that requires inspiration. Recommended balancing oils:

Suggestion Box

Here are oils and *Earth Tribe* blends to replenish our greatest natural resource—personal energy—which is too frequently in short supply.

1. Provides relief from stress and anxiety: lavender, geranium, *Calming Essential Oil*, *Calming Body Oil*, *Sweet Dreams, Love* (bath, perfume, diffuse)

2. Regulates mood/relieves depression: geranium, bergamot, orange, *Balance, Euphoria* (perfume, diffuse)

3. Stimulates mental activity/enhances memory: basil, peppermint, rosemary, *Head Peace* (diffuse, spray)

4. Invigorates and energizes: juniper, rosemary, *Energize* (diffuse)

5. Facilitates meditation/soothes: patchouli, sandalwood, *Recovery, Love, Prosperity* (perfume, diffuse, inhalation)

6. Entices romance: ylang-ylang, sandalwood, rose, *Night Fire Essential Oil Blend, Night Fire Massage Oil, Love, Volupté* (use in base spray, perfume, massage, bath)

bergamot, geranium, *Earth Tribe Balance* blend.

• Third chakra: Located in the solar plexus between the ribs and navel, this chakra acts as our guide to personal will, intention, and self-control. If you have trouble with commitment, temporarily or permanently, your third chakra is out of whack. No male jokes, please. Recommended balancing oils: juniper, basil, *Earth Tribe Energize* blend.

• Fourth chakra: Also known as the *heart chakra* for its location, it serves as the domain of human intimacy. Compassion blooms and grows here. Tibetan Buddhists believe "a compassionate heart is a victorious heart." Recommended balancing oils: rose, *Earth Tribe Love* blend.

• Fifth chakra: Called the *throat chakra*, the fifth chakra is actually located in the back of the neck and governs self-expression. Tending to it helps you find your true inner voice, which has to be one of the most wonderful results of any life-balancing effort. This is where your deepest truth can sometimes hide

Earth Healing
Karen Dudley

Karen Dudley had brain surgery about a year ago. The surgery resulted in postoperative injury. She soon started experiencing headaches, which she describes as "migrainelike."

After two months of suffering, Karen discovered the *Earth Tribe Head Peace* synergistic blend that features basil and rosemary essential oils. "It's working," says Karen. "The headaches were unexpected," she explains. "I am so glad to find a natural source of relief instead of pharmaceutical medications."

Nobody is more conscious about energy levels than athletes with serious intentions about their favorite sports and physical activities. So it makes perfect sense that essential oils can boost any athlete's training routine.

University of Alaska–Fairbanks researcher Anita Bush conducted a study of twenty men: those who relaxed in a room with lavender essential oil in a diffuser recovered significantly faster from a cardiovascular workout than those who relaxed in another room with no lavender. Blood pressure and heart rate for the first group returned to normal more rapidly. How you recover from a workout is a key indicator of fitness.

Here are some items you can start using with your next workout:

- Eucalyptus essential oil

This is an excellent option if you tend to get colds frequently. Think of it as preventive maintenance. It cools the body in summer and protects it in the winter. Use it as a disinfectant, an insect repellant, a decongestant, and for relief from sinus pain and sore muscles. You can rub it directly on the affected area or use in it a diffuser in your bedroom at night.

- *Peppermint* essential

Cooling after a workout or other strenuous activity. Use with base oil as an after-workout spray. Use also for muscle pain, digestive problems, bad breath, and headaches.

- *Muscle Soothe* synergistic blend

    A soothing *Earth Tribe* formulation designed to help alleviate the discomforts of overworked, overstressed muscles, strains and sprains, and sore muscles and joints. The main ingredients are sweet birch and peppermint essential oils. Apply topically.

- *Energize* synergistic blend

    Jumpstart your mornings and your workouts, or relieve afternoon energy lows and general fatigue with this stimulating blend. You can directly inhale it or apply it to your skin in the hour before you exercise. The main ingredients are juniper and peppermint essential oils.

- *Herbal Cooling Cream*

    An effective, soothing ointment for muscle soreness, injuries, strains and sprains, back pain, and tired aching muscles. The main ingredients are peppermint, lavender, and birch essential oils, the herb St. John's wort, and aloe vera.

- *Muscle Soothe Massage Oil*

    Relax and relieve discomfort in sore, tired muscles before or after strenuous activity—a great all-over body massage oil for the active. It seems to work best the sooner it is used after strenuous activity. The main ingredients are peppermint, sweet birch, Roman chamomile, and marjoram.

out or strengthen. Use plant oils for more of the latter and less of the former. Recommended balancing oils: eucalyptus, cedarwood, *Earth Tribe Breathe* blend.

• Sixth chakra: This chakra is known as the *third eye* because it originates between the eyebrows and governs our personal vision and ability to see truth in the world. Also plays a role in intuition, which, especially for women, is a big enough issue to warrant two chakras. Recommended balancing oils: rosemary, basil, *Earth Tribe Head Peace* blend.

• Seventh chakra: Right at the top of your head, this *crown chakra* focuses our attention on the spiritual meaning in life. It is a pivot point for the boundlessness we can feel in trusting a higher power. Indeed, heady stuff but most effectively felt in the heart and soul. So there, right-brained people! Recommended balancing oils: sandalwood, cedarwood, frankincense, *Earth Tribe Prosperity* blend.

• Eighth chakra: In some belief systems, such as kundalini yoga, the human form takes on its own overall chakra. It is identified as the invisible electromagnetic field surrounding our entire bodies. This radiance can extend up to nine feet from the body. This chakra might seem less tangible without an actual body point, but how many times have you heard someone talk about a person's magnetic personality or remarked how a bride was radiant on her wedding day. This chakra is most balanced when we believe in what we are doing or saying. Recommended balancing oils: rose, neroli, *Earth Tribe Glow* blend.

Chapter 5

Minding
Your Stress

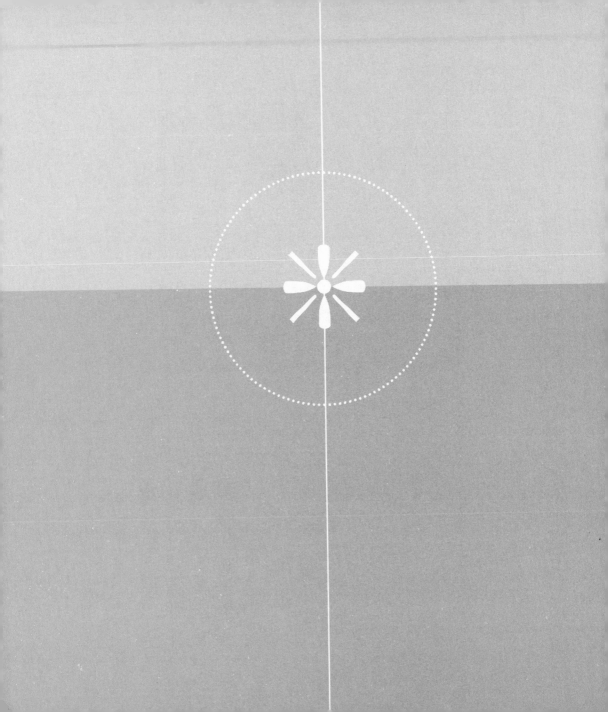

I can't tell you how many times stress becomes the main topic at essential oils seminars I lead. People feel stress in their bodies, brains, and—maybe most tellingly—souls. Their truest selves, which equates to their happiest selves, seem to slip away.

Researchers confirm the pattern. Studies about stress indicate that people who feel most burdened, most tired, most frazzled are those who feel they have the least amount of control in their lives. They don't feel they are living the life they want, nor can they say yes to the question, "Are your needs being met?"

One landmark study showed that British civil workers with relatively easy clerical jobs and little authority were more stressed than supervisors. Even if the managers were working harder and longer hours, they

Brain Break

There are some parallels between using essential oils and practicing yoga. In both cases, the mind-body-spirit breakthrough comes with slowing down the breathing. In a yoga class, you might begin with a meditation to get you in this state. And if you struggle during the opening meditation, chances are your mind will quiet down or empty as you concentrate on breathing during your postures (called *asanas*).

Using essential oils might take a bit more purposeful effort. Whenever you take a *brain break* by inhaling a plant oil from your diffuser or steaming container of water, be sure to breathe deeply. Concentrate solely on the breath; imagine inhaling into the bottom half of the lungs, where most Americans never reach. If your mind wanders, fine, let go of the thought and refocus on the breathing. Soon, your body and brain will naturally slow down together. And your mind gets a much needed rest; even a minute or two can work wonders.

The typical person takes twelve to fifteen breaths per minute. Your goal for a brain break is five to eight. When you become more attuned, you will know when your breathing is slow enough without even counting.

worried less because many decisions were in their hands. The clerical workers didn't have the same luxury and their health conditions suffered for it, especially over longer time periods.

Plant oils can't get you a promotion (at least not directly!) or instantly repair a relationship, but using them can give you back some sense of control. You can make your life feel more natural.

Better yet, essential oils can offset the stress that seems to come all too fast and furious in today's world. Aromatic molecules in plant essences reach the nose, then lock onto tiny receptors there to create electrical impulses through a tiny structure in the nose called the vomeronasal organ (VNO). Researchers are still exploring exactly how and if the VNO consistently sends signals to the brain about relaxing, feeling more confident, or gauging attraction to others. These impulses travel up the olfactory nerves to the brain, where the main destination is the limbic system. This region of the brain is where emotions and memory are processed.

The right oils can instruct the limbic system to send out messages for the body to slow down. The oils lead the brain to produce slower frequency brain waves (delta and theta waves). What's more, the oils prompt the brain to increase alpha brain waves, which help you feel centered and focused.

Psychology researchers are finding that essential plant oils can reduce apprehension, loneliness, and rejection, all of which have been linked to poor health. Loneliness, for instance, ancient as it might be, is considered a cutting-edge predictor of heart disease. Some oils used to offset negative feelings are bergamot, neroli, and Roman chamomile. You can use orange, jasmine, frankincense, and melissa to encourage positive feelings of solitude. Neroli and Roman chamomile do both.

Plant oils can actually make people less embarrassed or angry. One study asked participants, "What kind of person makes you angry?" then used pleasant scents with half of the group and nothing with the other half. People who inhaled pleasant scents calmed down significantly faster than the control group. Oils that can help you cope with anger

Earth Healing

Gurmukh

Her student roster reads like the invite list to an exclusive Oscars party, but Gurmukh Kaur Khalsa is a yoga pioneer and instructor who is about as grounded as a person can get. She has found the balance we all seek in life, and teaches it at her Goldenbridge Yoga Center in Los Angeles. Cindy Crawford, Madonna, Courtney Love, Rosanna Arquette, David Duchovny, members of the Red Hot Chili Peppers rock band, and many others have sought her insights—and don't want to miss her classes in Kundalini yoga, which emphasizes meditation and chanting along with a physical workout.

"I am aiming for people to find self-acceptance in their life," says Gurmukh, who is author of an inspiring new book, *The Eight Human Talents: The Yogic Way to Restore the Balance and Serenity Within You* (Cliff Street Books, 2000). "I am hoping that my students can stop always judging themselves."

(continued)

include lavender, rose, chamomile, vetiver, bergamot, ylang ylang, and patchouli. Try them in the bath.

Some essential oils, such as geranium and lavender, are called *adaptagens* because they can either stimulate or soothe the brain depending on circumstances. In both cases, I think the versatility—and stress-busting qualities—of these two oils proves the point that plants can provide powerful healing agents in our society without the nine-digit pharmaceutical advertising campaigns.

Researchers at such centers as the Smell and Taste Treatment and Research Foundation in Chicago and the Monell Chemical Senses Center in Philadelphia have found that our sense of smell provides the quickest route to changing mood and behavior for the better. It works faster than, say, meditating in silence, eating a delicious and healthy meal, seeing old friends, or holding hands with a loved one—even though I highly recommend each sensory activity.

Using plant oils might be just the ritual to establish at the time of day (kids in bed, workday done, phone stops ringing, kitchen cleaned up) when a glass of wine seems in order, to simply relax more deeply and completely. You may find you consume less alcohol. Our sense of smell is underrated and overlooked in its role as a stress-buster. Taking the step to make plant oils part of your everyday life can change all of that.

> ## Earth Healing *(continued)*
>
> Gurmukh uses essential oils and believes in their healing power. She sees them as one way to remind ourselves to practice "conscious breathing" and "quiet the mind." I am honored that she is a big fan of *Earth Tribe* essential oils. We had a terrific session the first time we met.
>
> "I liked Mary Lee's energy right away," Gurmukh told my coauthor Bob in an interview. "I feel she is sincere about making the world a better place, and her essential oils can help all of us find more balance and peace."

If using plant oils for stress doesn't entice you enough, or maybe you want to convince a stubborn loved one who thinks it is all some "nonsense about incense," then consider new research showing that the sense of smell can prevent Alzheimer's disease and other forms of memory loss. Premature loss of smell has been linked to Alzheimer's, and one study at Duke University showed that a smell test might be able to predict memory deterioration at earlier stages, when therapy can be most effective.

Your sense of smell is closely linked to the areas of the brain that

Mental Alert

Try these synergizing blends in your diffuser for alertness. It's easy as one, two, three.

1. Juniper (four drops)

   Lemon (two drops)

   Rosemary (two drops)

   or

2. Grapefruit (four drops)

   Black pepper (two drops)

   Peppermint (two drops)

   or

3. Eucalyptus (six drops)

   Peppermint (two drops)

   Basil (five drops)

control short- and long-term memory. Research indicates that people who inhale a scent while attempting to memorize a list of words have better retention later than individuals who used no scent while learning the list.

In fact, one researcher at Duke University, Lawrence C. Katz, has conducted a series of studies to make the case for using all five of our senses regularly and often to stave off memory loss and potential development of Alzheimer's. He says this full-sensory approach is many times more

Memorable Oils

These plant essences are ideal for improving alertness and focus:

Basil

Clove

Lemon

Rosemary

Balancing Act

Essential oils that stimulate alertness and memory can increase beta waves in the brain (see "Memorable Oils" list on this page), which can actually make some people feel more stressed. Rather than not use the oils, simply combine them with oils that balance your energy. Here are essential oils that have been tested favorably for producing a balanced effect. There is science behind the nature, folks.

Bergamot

Chamomile

Cedarwood

Lavender

Sandalwood

* Note: Although not tested in laboratories, these oils proved effective for the same relaxing reasons according to *Earth Tribe* clients: melissa (lemon balm), neroli (orange blossom), petitgrain, and rose.

No, I'm not going to say that a few drops of the proper plant oil will allow you to eat anything you want from french fries to fried ice cream. But I will say that research has proven certain scents can curb your appetite and cravings.When inhaled, essential oils travel to the brain's limbic system, which controls hunger. Plant oils, most notably sandalwood, can trigger certain neurochemicals in the brain that tell our bodies we are satisfied. So we eat less, reducing daily calorie intake and shedding unwanted pounds.

Earth Tribe has developed two specific *Slim Scents* formulas. One is called *Day Lite,* which features sandalwood and some of the brain-stimulating oils mentioned in this chapter. The other, *Night Lite,* curbs appetite and cravings but employs oils that calm the mind for rest.

There are several ways you can use *Slim Scents*. I especially recommend using it as a perfume or cologne or using it as your oil in aromatherapy jewelry (which are tiny containers that have holes for your oils to diffuse). You can also put *Slim Scents* or sandalwood oil into a base spray to spritz yourself or a room. Putting the oils in a diffuser or lightbulb ring are other good ideas.

We have studied the results of *Slim Scents* use by *Earth Tribe* customers. We found that individuals lost between five and fifteen pounds in four to eight weeks. Lynn Daly, who lives in Culver City, California, reported that she lost fourteen pounds in one month using our *Slim Scents* products.

"I carry the *Day Lite* with me everywhere I go. I am a mother of three young children, and I am extremely busy," says Daly. "*Day Lite* gives me the energy to get through the day while keeping my appetite under control.

"I was able to reduce my caloric intake, exercise on a consistent basis, and lose body fat. In the evening, I put *Night Lite* in my aroma lamp to set a calm, tranquil mood in our home. It prevented those nighttime munchies from getting me!"

Cellulite Patrol

Some oils can help with specific weight-related problems, such as dreaded cellulite. I strongly recommend using ten drops of grapefruit oil with an ounce of carrier oil for cellulite. Or you can use *Earth Tribe Slim-u-lite Massage Oil*, which is convenient and highly effective for lots of our customers. Massage on affected areas one to two times daily. You will notice the beginning of a difference within a week to ten days. Some customers report it happens even sooner. But be patient. The best results develop over several weeks to months. Just what results you can expect is a matter of how much cellulite you are hoping to eliminate. The first week to ten days should make a noticeable difference to the eye, and in two to four months, you are likely to feel significantly less self-conscious about the cellulite. Many *Earth Tribe* clients report clearing the problem completely within six months to a year. A good strategy is to use the oils as a preventive measure even once the cellulite has disappeared.

Confidence Boost

Here are some oils to use when your self-confidence needs a lift. My favorite blend is rosemary and basil, which are the active ingredients in the *Earth Tribe Head Peace* oil. It's a great blend for thinking positively:

Bergamot

Cedarwood

Ginger

Grapefruit

Jasmine

Orange

Rosemary

Sweet fennel

Vetiver

Good-News Oils

Orange, grapefruit, rose, clove, jasmine, ginger, geranium, and cinnamon are all terrific oils to encourage happiness or contentment. For a shot of pure joy, try sandalwood, bergamot, ylang ylang, petitgrain, chamomile, lemon, orange, neroli, or frankincense.

valuable to memory and overall brain function than mental engagement alone. For instance, he says playing bridge is preferable to working a crossword puzzle alone because the card game calls up all of the senses.

Research findings on the Philadelphia-based Monell Chemical Senses Center (Internet site www.monell.org) show that "odors are often thought to provide the best memory cues because some of our oldest and most emotionally laden memories are associated with odors. Accuracy of a memory is not affected by the type of sensory cue, whether it is olfactory or auditory, for example. Instead, a memory triggered by an odor is experienced as being more emotionally intense and evocative than a memory triggered by any other type of sensory cue."

Studies posted on the Web site also show that odors help people remember. "Memory is enhanced when learning takes place in the presence of a novel odor, and is further facilitated if learning occurs during a

Emptying the Water

If you have issues with water retention—and what woman doesn't?—try using your favorite application with juniper. Direct massage on the abdomen one to two times daily is a good strategy; use ten drops of juniper for every ounce of carrier oil for massage or ten drops in your bath water. Or you might opt for *Earth Tribe PMS Relief Rub*, which is good for all PMS symptoms. Diffusion is another effective method for cutting down on water retention, especially at key times in your menstrual cycle.

heightened emotional state," according to the Monell Center. I recommend keeping your office or work room scented with a diffuser or aromatherapy lightbulb ring for maximum productivity.

It's important to remember that essential oils are potent yet not intended to take the place of medicines prescribed by your doctor for a condition as serious as Alzheimer's or other measured memory loss. Clary sage, for instance, turns off the same enzymes in the brain to slow degeneration as some Alzheimer's drugs but at a lesser rate. On the other hand, clary sage doesn't tax the liver like these medications. Your best bet is to make essential oils a part of everyday life, which, of course, still includes regular visits to your health practitioner.

Chapter 6

Getting Chemicals out of Your Life— and Your Home

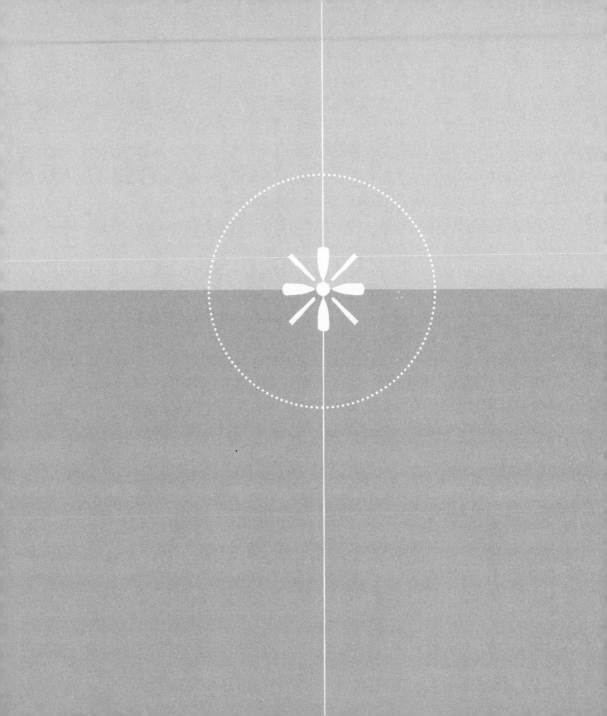

This is my favorite chapter.

Not because I love to clean house. Believe me I don't, though it is more satisfying and reassuring now that I use plant oils rather than harsh household cleaners. What makes me like this chapter so much is the huge difference plant oils can make in today's world simply by making them part of your daily cleaning routine. It can do wonders for your health, defeat pollution, and get your home cleaner all at the same time!

This book is not another in a long line about aromatherapy. If you get nothing else out of my Healthy Living program, I hope you do understand the importance of getting the chemicals out of our lives. Essential oils can help us replace potential toxins with effective alternatives and the home is a superb place to start.

Worrying about household chemicals is a relatively new preoccupation. Since World War II, there has been a petrochemical boom in this country and other industrialized nations. Companies realized these synthetic chemicals could be produced cheaply and in large quantities as active ingredients in household cleaners and personal hygiene products to kill germs and other microorganisms.

All of which sounds good enough, until you realize that petrochemicals don't discriminate between harmful bacteria and good bacteria or the flora that actually help our bodies fight off germs, infection, and other foreign invaders. The petrochemicals, which turn out to give us a false sense of security and cleanliness, disrupt our body's natural order of balance. I liken it to the old adage of throwing out the baby with the

Cleanup Hitter

Here's a lineup of quick tips for cleaning house with essential oils:

• Place a few drops of **lemon** (a natural bacteria-buster) down drains and disposals to clean, disinfect, and scent.

• Use **lavender** and **lemon** on a moist cloth and wipe down kitchen counters, bathroom tiles, showers, and tubs.

• Place a few drops of **lemon** on a piece of scrunched-up newspaper to polish windows (it also makes your home smell delightful when the sun shines on your windows).

• Spray linens, draperies, and furniture with *Earth Tribe*'s *Claire* to refresh and clean.

bathwater. And our kids are indeed most at risk. Our grandmothers and mothers could rely on safe all-around household cleaning and personal care products. But you, me, and especially today's children have all been increasingly exposed to synthetic petrochemicals. No one in history has faced the toxic experience confronting each of our children today.

The National Academy of Science estimates that 15 percent of Americans have chemical sensitivity that affects their quality of life. Experts only expect the number to rise—unless we do something about the chemicals in our lives.

There are approximately 70,000 chemicals now used in commercial products, up from practically none before World War II. Household cleaners contain about 4,000 toxic chemicals, which cause long-term nerve damage or death if ingested. The question, for which no one seems to know a definitive answer, is what damage those same chemicals do through everyday exposure to the skin and respiratory system.

I say let's not find out the hard way.

This monumental increase in household chemicals is one big reason why the U.S. Environmental Protection Agency (EPA) considers indoor air pollution one of this country's top five environmental threats. The EPA says air pollution inside the home can be two to five times higher— and occasionally even ten times higher—than air pollution outdoors.

Before the 2000–2001 school year, the largest organization of heating, air conditioning, and ventilation engineers, HVAC, issued a new report outlining the poor air quality of many school buildings (more than 8 million kids are exposed to unhealthy air). What's more, the HVAC specifically recommended being cautious about room deodorizer "plug-ins" that spray synthetic chemicals into the air. My guess is those same experts would be enthusiastic about diffusers and aroma lamps in classrooms as they provide the desired effect with all-natural components.

Yet one recent survey by the American Lung Association shows that nine out of ten Americans don't know about indoor air pollution. As our society begins using more herbs and other natural medicines, it only makes sense that cleaning up indoor air, home cleaners, and personal care products becomes the next step. Essential oils and *Earth Tribe* products can give you a head start.

Residues from more than 400 toxic chemicals, including a good number from household products, have been identified in human blood and fat tissue. The Consumer Product Safety Commission has determined that more than 150 chemicals in ordinary household cleaners have the potential to cause cancer, nerve system damage, birth defects, and fertility problems.

Some of the risk to children comes from innocent ingestion or extreme exposure of household cleaners and other products. Roughly 4,000 children each year are admitted to emergency rooms for household cleaner–related poisoning. Another 13,500 kids fourteen and under—and 4,500 adults—make trips to the emergency room for pesticide-related problems. What is equally scary about exposure among kids is that their smaller and still developing bodies are reacting to the chemicals in household products at higher levels.

In response, my company offers consumers safe, simple, and effective alternatives to potentially toxic household cleaners. But *Earth Tribe* and essential oils are not just for environmental extremists or the chemically sensitive anymore. Our plant oils and related products are for people who consider themselves informed, smart shoppers. My Healthy Living plan is for people who have decided to take an active, holistic, and natural approach to protecting and maintaining health among themselves and their families. And it is easier than you think.

Let's take a tour of your home, stopping in each room to make some suggestions about how to use plant oils—and get rid of synthetic chemicals. You will need these basic supplies to get the job done:

1. Essential oils of lemon, lavender, tea tree, orange, eucalyptus, and geranium
2. Baking soda
3. Liquid castile soap
4. White vinegar
5. Plant sprayer
6. Squirt bottles
7. Distilled or spring water
8. Hot water

Room by Room

The Kitchen

- Use orange or grapefruit in an aroma lamp or *Earth Tribe Base Spray* to freshen air and get rid of cooking odors.

- Add your favorite oil to natural dishwashing liquid. Or make your own dishwashing liquid with this recipe. You can lift your spirits and clean up at the same time!
  Use ten drops of lemon essential oil, ten drops lavender essential oil, and ten drops orange essential oil.

BASIC OVEN CLEANER

½ cup baking soda

½ cup liquid castile soap

Seven drops lemon essential oil

Seven drops eucalyptus essential oil

Five drops lavender essential oil

1 cup hot water

Directions: Preheat oven to 225°F, then turn off and leave the door open. Combine ingredients and pour into a spray bottle. Shake well. Spray on oven walls, wait 15–20 minutes, wipe off, and repeat if necessary.

KITCHEN SINK SCRUB

½ cup baking soda

⅛ cup white vinegar

Five drops lemon essential oil

Five drops orange essential oil

Directions: Combine all ingredients.

TUB AND SHOWER SCRUB

½ cup baking soda

Ten drops tea tree essential oil

Ten drops lavender essential oil

Ten drops geranium essential oil

Directions: Combine all ingredients. Use with damp sponge or cloth to scrub shower and tub. Prevents mold and mildew buildup. For serious mildew buildup, combine twenty drops of tea tree oil and water in a small spray bottle; spray the area every day for five days, then twice a week.

Fill a twenty-eight- or thirty-two-ounce squirt bottle with castile soap, add the oils, and shake well before each use.

• For an instant natural disinfectant, put a few drops of orange, grapefruit, or our *Euphoria* blend (bergamot and orange) on a cloth moistened with water for wiping your countertops, tables, stove top, and other "hot spots" in the kitchen. Or try this recipe for an all-purpose disinfectant and countertop cleaner:

Use five drops of lavender essential oil, five drops of lemon essential oil, five drops of orange essential oil, five drops of eucalyptus essential oil, and five drops of tea tree essential oil.

Fill a small plant sprayer with water and add the oils.

On the Menu

Here are some ideas for adding certain essential oils to your food:

• Try adding two to three drops of orange into your cheesecake recipe, seasoned rice, cakes, cookies, or chicken. Remember: The oils are very potent. One or two drops replaces one teaspoon of herb or spice. Great for party punches also.

• Pierce a roasting chicken with a fork a few times, then sprinkle several drops of essential oil of rosemary onto the chicken before baking. Serve with fresh rosemary.

• When grilling fresh fish, sprinkle a few drops of essential oil of lemon on it.

Remember: Essential oils are very potent, much more potent than the herb or spice, so use it sparingly!

• Put a few drops of orange, lemon, and grapefruit down drains and disposal occasionally to clean and freshen. For distinct odors, use about eight drops while running disposal with water.

• Spray *Earth Tribe's All Natural Insect Repellant* around windows and floorboards to keep ants and other pests away.

The Bathroom

• Put a few drops of your favorite oil on the cardboard tube inside a roll of toilet paper to scent the room.

- For health and mood enhancement, add eight to ten drops of essential oil or essential oil blend to your bath.

- Combine six to ten drops total of lemon, orange, or grapefruit oil per pint of water for washing the floor and porcelain. For tough spots, apply oil directly to a wet cloth. Or you can use *Earth Tribe Claire* spray or other oils in a blend. Adjust for your own cleaning challenges to which oil smells best to you and your family.

The Bedroom

- For a romantically scented bedroom, place thirty to forty drops of *Night Fire* (our blend featuring ylang ylang and clove oils) in *Earth Tribe Base Spray*. Spray bed linens and scent the air.

- For a great-smelling closet, moisten cotton balls with the *Breathe* blend (cedarwood, fir, eucalyptus, and pine) and place on closet shelves and drawers. The result is just like having a cedar closet! It helps keep the moths away, too.

- *Night Fire Body Oil* makes a wonderful massage oil for couples.

The Living Room

- Moisten a cotton ball with your favorite oil and place in a vacuum-cleaner bag to scent carpets and the air.

- Freshen furniture, curtains, carpet, and air with *Earth Tribe Base Spray,* to which you'll add thirty to forty drops of your favorite oil (orange and geranium are a wonderful combination, or use *Earth Tribe's Claire*).

- Use a clay pot diffuser or a nebulizing diffuser to create an atmosphere. Try these blends: *Calming* (lavender, chamomile) for family evenings; *Energize* (juniper, peppermint) for morning jump-starts; *Euphoria* (orange, bergamot) for entertaining; *Love* (ylang ylang, rose) for Valentine's Day and romantic interludes (get those kids to bed!); and lavender and orange for children's parties.

The Laundry Room

- Moisten unscented dryer sheets or Handi-Wipes with your favorite oil (artificially scented dryer sheets are a major cause of skin rashes). Doing so helps make clothes germ-free and fragrant while protecting against mold and mildew in the dryer. Add a few drops to your wash as well!

The Home Office/Desk

- Scent stationery, business cards, notepads, and the like by putting a few drops of oil onto blotter paper. Place the blotter paper and whatever you wish to scent in a tightly closed box. Let it sit for one week. Or simply spray your papers with *Earth Tribe Base Spray* (to which you've added your favorite oil) and let them dry.

- Keep a spray bottle of *Claire* handy for air freshening. Its active ingredients are tea tree, eucalyptus, and lavender essential oils. You can spritz your desk chair a couple of times a week. Use a diffuser or spray bottle to scent the air with our *Prosperity* blend (frankincense, myrrh).

Playrooms/Children's Bedrooms

- Spray *Claire* all around to freshen the air and disinfect. It combats germs and cleans at the same time. It also smells good!
- *Monster Mist* sprayed in a child's room at night helps to calm and soothe.

Away from Home

- Take a travel-sized bottle of *Claire* for spraying airplane seats, hotel rooms, or even children's hands to clean and kill germs. Or add five drops each of lavender, lemon, orange, eucalyptus, and tea tree essential oils to a small spray bottle of water.

Don'ts and Do's

Here are some essential oil and other *Earth Tribe* alternatives to more harsh household cleaners:

All-Purpose Cleaners

Instead of using . . .

- 409
- Mr. Clean
- Fantastik
- ammonia

Get the Right Equipment

We aromatherapists have a term known as *environmental fragrancing*. It may sound fancy, but all it refers to is to keep the air as clean, fresh, and mood-enhancing as possible. While you can drop essential oil into a steaming container of water for therapeutic effect, here are some tools of the trade I strongly recommend purchasing for maximum benefit from your plant oils. Each of these items is a small investment (twenty-five dollars or less) for a big payoff:

NEBULIZING DIFFUSER

A forced-air, no-heat diffuser, such as *Earth Tribe's Nebulizing Diffuser* maximizes the therapeutic effect of any essential oil. For more information on nebulizers, see page 40.

CLAY POT DIFFUSER

These pottery diffusers are just right for smaller rooms—plus your automobiles and office cubicles. Put twenty to thirty drops of an essential oil or blend directly into the top of the bowl. The oils diffuse slowly through the terra-cotta, which is only glazed on the bottom. Get several for your personal spaces.

TERRA-COTTA LIGHTBULB RINGS

Place your lightbulb ring atop a standard lightbulb. Add eight to twelve drops of essential oil or blend to the inner rim. The room will quickly fill with natural fragrance.

EARTH TRIBE BASE SPRAY

Our all-natural, water soluble *Earth Tribe Base Spray* facilitates the use of essential oils and blends as a room spray/air freshener or body spray. Place thirty to fifty drops of essential oil or blend into the *Base Spray*. Shake well and spray your environment (home, office, car, etc.) or yourself. A natural way to disinfect the air or freshen yourself.

CANDLES AND INCENSE

These two methods are easy ways to distribute the natural healing powers of essential oils. Make sure the products you buy use pure oils and not synthetic materials or other "stretch" ingredients. You need the real thing to get the real benefits. And make sure the candle is made of natural waxes, such as vegetable wax and beeswax.

Moms and dads might want to be most careful about using home and garden pesticides. Statistics show the risk for leukemia increases four to seven times among children whose parents use such products. Other studies show an increased risk for brain cancer is associated with pesticide bombs in the home, pet flea collars, garden insecticides, and herbicides to kill weeds. Look for DEET as an active ingredient, then avoid that product. DEET is a hazardous chemical found to cause severe allergic reactions and even death.

Many of the active ingredients in these products are coming under tighter review by the government, but there is still much controversy. Insect repellants are especially worrisome to enlightened parents I meet at *Earth Tribe* seminars and other functions. Here are some essential-oil alternatives that can work for you—and that smell infinitely much better than any pesticide or insect repellant! I know they are effective because I have tried them at home with my twin boys underfoot.

• You can make your own skin-safe natural insect repellant by adding about ten drops of eucalyptus and five each of cedarwood and sandalwood to two ounces of rubbing alcohol (or even vodka if you can believe it). Store it in a glass container. Some aromatherapists recommend adding citronella or pennyroyal oils to the mix, but both can be hazardous for pregnant women. Citronella candles are alternatives. Another strategy is to add a few drops of the pleasantly aromatic geranium oil, which in itself has some bug-repelling qualities. In any case, remember that natural oils are potent; don't use repellant and then immediately wipe your mouth or eyes.

- If you don't want to make your own, *Earth Tribe All Natural Plant Essence Insect Repellant* will keep mosquitoes at bay (and it's even safe for babies). I created it when the twins were six months old and I made my first trek back home to northern Minnesota. The natural repellant contains sandalwood, cedarwood, and eucalyptus, which are oils that have been used by Native Americans for centuries. It also works exceptionally well in the home to keep ants, flies, gnats, and other insects away. Spray wherever you see ants, especially at their point of entry. Our repellant is perfectly safe for babies and children, and even makes a great skin moisturizer.

- To keep pests out of the garden, place twenty to forty drops of peppermint in *Earth Tribe Base Spray*, then mist your plants. Or you can add the oils while watering your garden.

- For fleas, use orange, eucalyptus, or peppermint in an aroma lamp or *Earth Tribe Base Spray*.

Try these alternatives . . .

- lemon essential oil
- grapefruit essential oil
- tea tree essential oil
- *Earth Tribe Claire*

How to use: Place ten to twelve drops of oil on a moist cloth. Use six to ten drops per pint of water for washing floors. Use *Claire* as an all-purpose cleaning/disinfecting spray.

Glass Cleaner

Instead of using . . .

- Glass Plus
- Windex

Try these alternatives . . .

- grapefruit essential oil
- lemon essential oil
- *Earth Tribe Euphoria*

How to use: Scrunch up a piece of newspaper and use seven to ten drops of oil or *Euphoria* to polish windows and glass. It will create a pleasant scent when the sun shines on the windows. You can also use paper towels, though the less absorbent the better.

Drain Cleaners

Instead of using . . .

- Mr. Clean
- Liquid Plumber
- Drano

Try these alternatives . . .
- lemon essential oil
- *Earth Tribe Euphoria*

How to use: Put ten to fifteen drops down the drain, wait one minute, then run warm water.

Floor Cleaners/Polishers
Instead of using . . .
- Pine-Sol
- Step Saver
- Mop and Glo

Try these alternatives . . .
- eucalyptus essential oil
- lemon essential oil

How to use: For linoleum and tile floors, combine six tablespoons of cornstarch, one cup of water, and ten drops of oil in a bucket. For wood floors, combine one cup of white vinegar, ⅛ cup of liquid castile soap, and twenty drops of above oils in two gallons of warm water.

Air Fresheners/Deodorizers

Instead of using . . .

- Glade aerosols
- Renuzit air fresheners
- Glade plug-ins
- Glade country pottery

Try these alternatives . . .

- Nebulizing diffuser
- Lightbulb ring
- Clay pot diffuser
- *Earth Tribe Base Spray*

How to use: Place about thirty to fifty drops of your favorite essential oil in the *Earth Tribe Base Spray*. Or place six to twelve drops in the aroma lamp, eight to twelve in the lightbulb ring, or twenty to thirty drops in the diffuser.

Cleansers

Instead of using . . .

- Ajax
- Comet

Try these alternatives . . .

- lemon essential oil, lavender essential oil, and tea tree essential oil
- *Euphoria* blend and tea tree essential oil

How to use: Mix ten drops of essential oil in ½ cup of baking soda and use it to scour and scrub.

Insect Repellants

Instead of using . . .

- Off!
- Black Flag
- Raid

Try these alternatives . . .

- peppermint essential oil
- *Earth Tribe All Natural Insect Repellant*

How to use: Use oils indoors to drive away ants and other household pests simply by spraying counters, floors, and wherever bugs might be. These are safe for use around babies and pets.

Garden Pesticides

Instead of using . . .

- Combat
- Black Flag Garden

Try these alternatives . . .

- lavender essential oil
- peppermint essential oil

How to use: Add the oils to water when spraying your plants or garden. Or you can place a few drops directly on the affected plants. Do not use

Earth Healing

Brian Danelian

From baby to beard, Brian Danelian is a happy *Earth Tribe* customer. He first learned about essential oils when his infant son, Dominic, was having trouble sleeping and, at times, breathing. Brian and his wife, Andrea, used *Earth Tribe Lullabye Baby Rub* on Dominic's tummy to help with colic. "It really did help," says Brian, a financial advisor who lives in Sherman Oaks, California. "We use all of the *Earth Tribe* products for Dominic's bath. My wife swears by them [for both Dominic and his four-year-old sister, Ariana]." Brian keeps a bottle of face oil for himself, and uses it to maintain his goatee in top style. "Otherwise, it can get very dry and flaky," says Brian. "The face oil is phenomenal. I use it every morning."

peppermint oil with tropical plants.

Animal Instincts

Making your household more natural can include family pets, too. Aromatherapy and the use of essential oils can be a perfect choice for your pet. There is a Native American belief that we are all related—plant kingdom, animal kingdom, and humans. We borrow wisdom and learn from one another.

I know I would much rather use something on my body, in my home, on my children, and on my pets that has evolved right alongside this human system for thousands of years than something that was made or created in a lab last month, or even in the last decade! By using essential oils and aromatherapy we are borrowing wisdom from the plant kingdom, and who knows, maybe it was the animals that first taught us to look to the plant kingdom for health and healing.

Animals instinctively know how to heal themselves and what plants to eat, rub up against, or lie down among when they are ill. Perhaps if we observe more closely the exchange between animals and plants, we humans will benefit greatly.

I have seen firsthand the amazing effects that essential oils have on pets. The pet owners who use my essential oil products are happy to report that their pets feel more comforted, have more balance and natural vitality, and seem happier. Actresses Natassja Kinski, Jami Gertz, and Jennie Garth are all concerned pet owners that use my formulations!

We have found various ways that pets are healthier and happier when essential oils are incorporated into their care:

- reduced "pet odors" and better hygiene
- healthier coat and skin
- pain relief
- insects kept away naturally
- first aid
- calming and comforting
- bonding
- more effective training sessions

The methods of application for pets are the same as for humans.

1. Through inhalation:
- diffuse into the air
- spray into the air
- place on cloth or blanket
- wear as a perfume (owners and trainers)

PET FRESH SPRAY

Into one cup of purified water add:

- ten drops of essential oil of lavender
- five drops of essential oil of orange
- five drops of essential oil of Roman chamomile

Place water and essential oils together in a sprayer and mist your pet and the pet's sleeping area.

ALL-NATURAL INSECT REPELLANT

Into ½ cup of vegetable oil add:

- twenty drops of essential oil of lavender
- thirty drops of essential oil of orange
- five drops of essential oil of eucalyptus
- five drops of essential oil of peppermint

Mix together in a sprayer and spray on your pet's coat and in sleeping area.

ALL-PURPOSE BOOBOO JUICE

Into a bowl of warm water add:

- ten drops of essential oil of lavender
- ten drops of essential oil of tea tree
- two drops of essential oil of orange

Saturate a cloth with this mixture and place it gently on the injured area.

MUSCLE AND JOINT SOOTHER

Into one cup of vegetable or nut oil add:

- twenty drops of essential oil of peppermint
- ten drops of essential oil of Roman chamomile
- ten drops of essential oil of eucalyptus
- twenty drops of essential oil of vetiver

ANTI-ITCH SPRAY

Into one cup of purified water add:

- twenty drops of essential oil of lavender
- twenty drops of essential oil of peppermint
- twenty drops of essential oil of tea tree

Put essential oils and water together in a sprayer and spray affected areas.

Note: Always use essential oils with caution and avoid eyes, nose, and genitals. Dilute before applying oils directly to the skin.

2. Through the skin:
- massage
- bath and shampoo
- direct topical application
- spray mists
- compresses
- grooming

The following essential oils are invaluable when something quick and effective is needed for your pets:

- Lavender: calming and great for nervousness, and for cuts, scrapes, hot spots, insect bites, burns
- Tea tree: antifungal; conditions paws and claws; fights viral infections
- Orange: insect repellant, mood elevator, air purifier
- Eucalyptus: insect repellant; fights colds and respiratory congestion

Chapter 7

An Antidote for Antibiotics

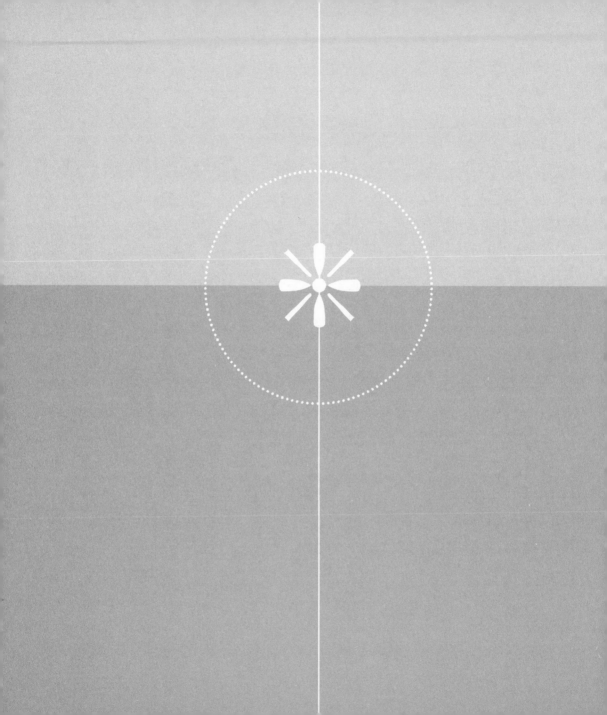

It's not overly important

to know exactly where Healthy Living leaves off and Natural Health begins in my Healthy Living plan. Using essential oils is all about developing a healthier lifestyle, or what I call an improved *healthstyle*.

But what is critical is knowing when you have slipped from a natural healthstyle to one that depends on synthetic chemicals. Far too many Americans rely on prescription drugs and over-the-counter medications as their remedies for minor illnesses. Plant oils provide a safe, effective option that can return us to natural health rather than depend on artificial intelligence.

The best example (or you might say worst) of our unnatural ways is the overuse of antibiotics in this country. The U.S. Centers for Disease Control and Prevention (CDC) estimates half of the 100 million prescriptions for antibiotics written by doctors every year are unnecessary. More shocking, 25 million of those prescriptions are written for viral infections such as colds, flu, and viral bronchitis despite the fact antibiotics have absolutely no effect on viruses.

Sorry to say it, but there is an even bigger problem with antibiotic use. You probably have heard about antibiotic resistance. An antibiotic drug is one that kills or inhibits the growth of bacteria, which is good. But taking an antibiotic when you don't need it—such as when the problem is a viral infection or you have a mild bacterial infection that will run its limited course within days—only gives other bacteria in your body the chance to scout the drug. The weaker bacteria and germs are killed off, but the bacteria with more evolved defense systems actually develop and colonize strains that can resist the drug next time it enters the body. Plus, there are newer studies showing that these superbacteria can actually pass on their resistance to other bacteria that have never encountered the drug.

Antiwellness

While antibiotics can clear bacterial infections, they come with a price. Side effects from antibiotics commonly include indigestion, yeast infections, and caffeine jitters. Some medications can make you highly sensitive to the sun. Medical journal case studies have even reported that one common antibiotic can weaken tendons, and thus cause torn Achilles tendons.

Over time these super bacteria aren't bothered by old standby antibiotics that have been used for decades to wipe out bacterial infections of the ears, sinuses, throat, lungs, blood, intestines, and urinary tract. As a result, illnesses last longer, become increasingly severe, and cost more to treat, and certain antibiotics are rendered useless. The medical community reaction? It has traditionally been to get pharmaceutical companies to make stronger antibiotics. That is starting to change. Along with the CDC, the National Institutes of Health, the American Medical Association, and the American Academy of Pediatrics have all called for a reappraisal and overhaul of how doctors and patients use antibiotics in this country.

When I first started studying essential oils, very few people seemed worried about antibiotic resistance or even knew it was a potential public health threat. But Dr. Andrew Weil, director of the pioneering integrative medicine program at the University of Arizona and best-selling

Now Ear This

Treating kids with antibiotics for frequent ear infections is practically a national pastime during the cold-weather months. But studies show the typical ten-day course of antibiotics used for childhood ear infections generally doesn't work. About 80 percent of kids don't get better any sooner with drugs. On the other hand, antibiotics can lead to vomiting or diarrhea, not to mention that your child might become resistant to antibiotics when he or she really needs them.

author, has voiced his concerns since his first book, *The Natural Mind*, was published in the early 1970s. "If we continue to use antibiotics as a cure-all," he says, "they will eventually become a cure-nothing."

In his writings and teachings, Dr. Weil calls for a drastically more conservative use of antibiotics by both doctors and patients (who ask for them routinely and sometimes don't want to leave the office without a prescription in hand to "solve" their problem). He also suggests a daily tonic made with an extract of the herb astragulus during the cold and flu season, plus eating foods with "probiotics," which are helpful bacteria found most prominently in yogurt, kefir, and fresh sauerkraut. If you feel yourself getting a cold or scratchy throat, Weil recommends taking an extract of echinacea to reduce symptoms and shorten the length of the illness.

Of course, he endorses getting plenty of fluids and rest, and, wisely, if pain or fever persists for more than three days, consulting your health practitioner. Weil is a leader among physicians who encourage patients to allow their bodies time to heal. As it turns out, by taking less antibiotics you give your immune system the opportunity to do some "cataloging" of its own. Your body generates the invader bacteria and makes its own cells to fight back. It clears the infection and is even better prepared to squash it next time.

I might humbly add to Weil's antidote for antibiotics. Plant oils can help your body defend its turf—and then some. Some essential oils are strong antibacterial agents, such as lavender, cinnamon, and thyme, among others (see Chart 7.1). Kansas State University researchers have discovered that ground cinnamon can kill dangerous bacteria in raw meat, such as E. coli; they found similar properties in extracts and powders of cloves, oregano, and sage. Other studies show that thyme oil is as

Branded

If you hesitate to jump with both feet into this essential oil thing—and remember I always recommend one step at a time—then you might want to check out the ingredients in longtime bacteria-fighter remedies. For instance, that leading brand-name aromatic chest rub your mom likely spread across your chest as a youngster got its kick from antibacterial compounds in eucalyptus, thyme, and mint. Or that top market-share mouthwash with the American Dental Association seal of approval for killing germs and plaque that cause gum disease, tooth decay, and bad breath? Its active agent was once thyme, plus some eucalyptus and mint. Now the mouthwash maker uses an alcohol compound, which is radically less expensive than thyme essential oil.

But—and this is important—thyme oil is such a strong antiseptic that it might burn sensitive skin. Better to use it in a prepared salve, and never apply it directly to the skin.

powerful as standard antibiotic drugs for killing intestinal bugs and lung infections such as staph and strep.

Best of all, the complex chemistry of essential oils—with untold phyto compounds in every molecule—makes it impossible for bacteria to develop a resistance. While harmful bacteria eventually overcome antibiotic medications, they can't do the same with plant oils. Although I like to think of my Healthy Living plan as simple to follow, this is one case that I welcome the complexity!

Chart 7.1. Natural Antibiotics

These essential oils are the most potent for killing harmful bacteria but not disturbing the "good" bacteria or flora in your body. They are strong bacteria killers, but be careful when using them to avoid burning the skin or mucous membranes.

- Cinnamon
- Clove bud
- Garlic
- Oregano
- Thyme

These oils are more gentle than those listed above, but they can still do the job. They are easier on the skin, and so generally safer to use.

- Eucalyptus
- Frankincense
- Geranium
- Helichrysum
- Lavender
- Lemon
- Lemongrass
- Manuka
- Marjoram
- Myrrh
- Pine
- Rose

- Sandalwood
- Sweet orange
- Tea tree
- Vetiver

Other essential oils are strong antiviral agents, actually making them more effective than antibiotics (which kill only bacteria, not viruses or fungi). Some natural antivirals, such as tea tree and manuka essential oils, are *triple-threats* that can kill bacteria, viruses, and fungi with each single drop. Other triple-threats include lavender, lemon, myrrh, and sage (see Charts 7.1, 7.2, and 7.3).

Tea tree is a strong and effective all-purpose healing oil. Just ask anyone who has used it to fight off a cold or beat athlete's foot. Tea tree essential oil originates with the Aborigine people who are native to Australia (and about whom we heard so much during the 2000 Summer Olympics in Sydney). The British explorer Captain John Cook actually named the tree because he noticed the Aborigines seemed to always be drinking tea brewed from its leaves.

Manuka essential oil is less known here in the United States, but I am excited to report that *Earth Tribe* is now using it in some products, including in our *Cold and Flu Rub*. It has long been a staple of the Maori tribes in New Zealand (Polynesian people who migrated to New Zealand in canoes) and the secret is about to get out worldwide. You can say you read it here first. Manuka essential oil appears to boost the healing properties of tea tree oil when the two are used together. Gotta love that synergy!

Chart 7.2. Natural Antivirals

These essential oils can fight viruses, which is not something you can say about antibiotic drugs.

- Bergamot
- Eucalyptus
- Geranium
- Lavender
- Lemon
- Lemongrass
- Manuka
- Melissa
- Rose
- Rosemary
- Sage
- Tea tree

These oils fight viral infections. When using them, be careful to avoid harming the skin or mucus membranes.

- Cinnamon
- Clove bud
- Garlic
- Oregano
- Thyme

Happily, a good number of essential plant oils can neutralize fungal infection. Once a fungus takes hold, it can spread quickly. It can itch like

Cold Wars

One of the best things you can do for yourself and your family is to use plant oils to treat common colds and flu. These viruses won't be quelled by antibiotics and modern medicine hasn't figured out any other foolproof way to stop them. An antiviral oil is actually your best defense. Here are some ideas for fighting colds more naturally, safely, and effectively:

• Use a few drops of a natural antiviral (see Chart 7.2) in steaming water, then inhale it deep into your sinuses and lungs. **Important: Don't use oregano, black pepper, cinnamon, or garlic essentials in this method; they are concentrated and hot enough to cause a burning sensation.**

• For cold sores, herpes, and other viral skin infections, use a salve or lip balm with a natural antiviral. Or make your own with five drops in a half-ounce of carrier oil (almond, jojoba, avocado, grapeseed, or even olive).

• Give yourself a chest and neck massage with *Earth Tribe Cold and Flu Rub* (active ingredients are tea tree, manuka, lavender, and eucalyptus essential oils).

• Put lavender and tea tree or *Earth Tribe Breathe* blend (eucalyptus and fir essential oils) in a bath. Eight to ten drops for adults, two to five for kids.

• Put six to twelve drops of a natural antiviral in a diffuser or humidifier for overnight breathing. Try a blend of eucalyptus, tea tree, and lavender.

• Place two drops of lavender or *Earth Tribe Breathe* on your pillow at night. Or you can scent a cotton ball with two drops of oil and position it under the edge of your pillow. Safe for babies and children.

• In more than a footnote, you can put essential oils in your bedsocks to help clear a cold or flu. Take a piece of tissue, tear it in two, and put a couple of drops of a natural antiviral on each piece of tissue. Then place a piece inside each sock so that it sits flat against the sole.

Caution: Remember that some infections are not to be underestimated. If pain, fever, or extreme fatigue lasts more than three days, make sure to see a health practitioner. For instance, pneumonia is either a bacterial or viral infection that needs close attention to avoid serious consequences, including death. Essential oils can help you recover, but this is a time when modern medicine can shine. Bacterial pneumonia is more serious but can be effectively treated with antibiotics.

crazy and can pass from one person to another rather easily. Fingernails, toenails, and feet are typical trouble spots. Soaking in a hand- or footbath that includes a few drops of a natural antifungal essential oil (see Chart 7.3) is effective.

If you have a mouth infection that is described by patchy splotches, it's likely you have candida or a yeast infection. Try swabbing the inside of your mouth with a Q-tip dipped in one or two drops of natural antifungal diluted in vegetable oil. For vaginal yeast infections, women can use one or two drops of tea tree essential oil (not black pepper, cinnamon, clove, or peppermint, all of which can burn) in plain yogurt as a douche.

One more pointer: Whether you use an essential oil preparation to fight bacteria, viruses, or funguses—or all three—repeat the application every several hours to maintain a constant level of the plant's natural healing agents. This is especially true for an acute (but still relatively minor) condition. If your condition is serious or lasts more than three days without improvement, don't hesitate to consult your health practitioner.

Excuse me if I repeat myself, but I want you to understand that I am not a doctor and don't presume to offer medical advice. What I am is a patient much like you who happens to have a lot of experience with these natural remedies. I want to take as few drugs as possible, and I think the world will be a better and healthier place if more people make that pledge. I have kids and don't want them taking medications unnecessarily. I want them to grow up recognizing the healing power of essential oils. My hope for them is to live in a world less influenced by chemicals.

Chart 7.3. Natural Antifungals

These essential oils fight funguses effectively yet gently.

- Bergamot
- Fennel
- Geranium
- Lavender
- Lemon
- Manuka
- Marjoram
- Melissa
- Rosemary
- Tea tree

Earth Healing

Catherine Johnson

Doesn't it seem like our bodies always give out just when we are about to go on vacation? Proponents of the mind-body connection would speculate that the mind signals the body to relax a bit too much and we catch a cold or flu. Others would contend most people simply cram a lot of work into the final days before a vacation, and then pile on the usual packing and other preparation for taking a trip.

But no matter which side you take about why we get sick, Catherine Johnson, a California massage therapist, is inclined to be proactive about avoiding a full-blown illness and fully blown vacation.

"I recently came down with a cold just a day before a scheduled vacation to London," says Johnson, who uses essential oils with her clients. "I was rather alarmed since I knew that a ten-hour trip in a pressurized cabin would be uncomfortable with congestion. I sprayed the

(continued)

These oils are all good fungus-fighters, but be careful about using them directly on the skin or mucous membranes. They can burn.

- Basil
- Cinnamon
- Clove bud
- Oregano
- Peppermint
- Thyme

Triple Threats

These essential oils are effective in fighting bacteria, viruses, and funguses—all in each drop! They are gentle enough to use for skin preparations (neat or in carrier oil) directly on the skin.

- Lavender
- Lemon
- Manuka
- Marjoram
- Myrrh
- Tea tree

These oils also fight all three types of infections, but use them with caution—always greatly diluted in carrier oils—because their potency can inadvertently burn the skin or mucous membranes.

- Cinnamon
- Clove bud
- Oregano
- Thyme

Double Duty Chart

These oils are effective in treating both bacteria and viruses. The ones marked with an asterisk also fight funguses. The whole list can be handy when you have an infection but aren't sure if it is bacterial or viral (sinus congestion is a prime example).

- Eucalyptus
- Geranium
- Lavender*
- Lemon*
- Marjoram*
- Myrrh*
- Rose
- Tea tree*

Earth Healing (continued)

Earth Tribe Breathe blend on myself, in the air around me, on my seat, and applied it directly to the temples and nasal passages.

"Not only was my congestion tremendously relieved, but I was able to enjoy long sightseeing days with little congestion or symptoms. I was so impressed with the product's results, I recommended it to a client who flies transcontinental several times a month and who suffers from chronic sinusitis. She thinks it's a miracle."

Traditional Menus

We can learn something about the hot topic of food safety from cultural traditions. They understood that spices help keep food from spoiling, while fighting bacteria in the process. Paul Sherman, a biologist at Cornell University in Ithaca, New York, examined more than 4,100 traditional recipes from thirty-six cultures. What he found was that people who lived in hotter climates consumed spicier foods.

So Sherman tested forty-three spices for their ability to control and kill off thirty different kinds of bacteria that can be detrimental to foods. Onion, garlic, oregano, and allspice knocked out all thirty invaders, while cumin, cinnamon, cloves, and cayenne peppers eliminated more than twenty each.

Other research shows that essential oils of bay, cinnamon, thyme, and clove were the most potent among twenty-one oils tested for destroying common sources of food poisoning such as E. coli, salmonella, listeria, and staphylococcus. Of course, you shouldn't ingest essential oils. So adding these spices and herbs to your recipes in available edible forms (dried or fresh) makes it easy to get these health-boosters into your digestive system. And chances are your food will taste better!

Chapter 8

No Kidding
Around

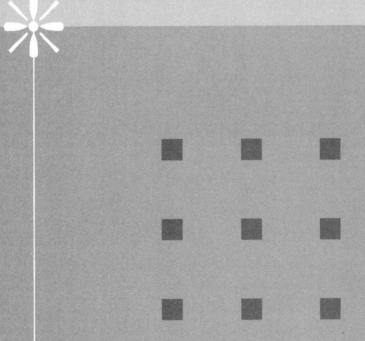

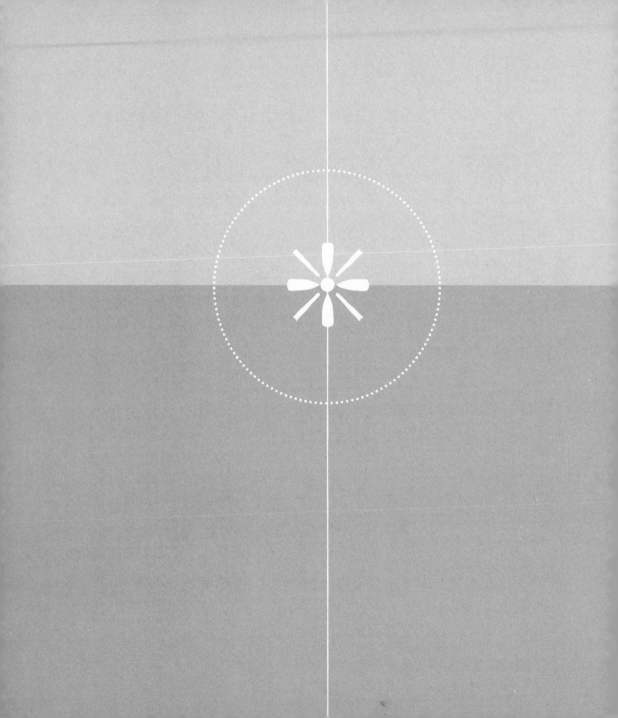

Imagine you are a first-time mother just home from the hospital with your precious child. So many questions arise each day about your baby's care and well-being. The time comes for your baby's first bath at home.

You reach for a commercial brand of soap, perhaps one you think of as mild, say, Ivory. You read the label with a whole new perspective: sodium cocoyl isethionate, paraffin, sodium cocoglyceryl ether sulfonate, stearic acid, sodium chloride, lauric acid, titanium dioxide, and trisodium etidronate. Those are just some of the twenty-two chemicals listed as ingredients in a brand advertised as *pure*. It sounds more like a science experiment or maybe substances for rocket fuel.

You start thinking, there must be a better way.

Earth Healing

B. J. Perkins

He was no different than many teenagers, or so it might have seemed. B. J. Perkins just couldn't be still or quiet, whether in the classroom or in his own bed at night. His motor kept revving up even when his mind rested.

The hyperactivity was affecting more than B.J.'s grades, which were progressively worse each semester because of his inability to concentrate. His main personality trait was irritability and a good night's sleep was no more realistic than a hundred imaginary sheep dancing overhead. At sixteen, the teen was at his wit's end.

His mother was equally distraught. She took her son to the best sleep disorder clinics and to physicians who specialized in learning problems. Nothing seemed to work, including potent prescription drugs.

B.J.'s mom decided to try the *Earth Tribe Sweet Dreams* synergistic blend, which combines essential oils of lavender and marjoram.

(continued)

There is, and nature provides it. Essential oils can bathe your baby, soothe a child's cuts, boost kids' energy and moods, and nurse the family through the cold and flu season—all effectively and without any artificial ingredients or fallout from synthetic chemicals.

I got started studying essential oils because it healed my severe burns, but it became a mission for me because of my twin boys, Talor and Micah, who turned eight on December 30, 2000. When I first took them home I was determined to not use any synthetic chemicals with them if I could help it.

That would include everything from avoiding toxins in the home to taking too many antibiotics and other medications to eliminating the chemicals we use for everyday first-aid and comfort.

My no-chemicals vow required lots of hours in my kitchen attempting new blends and recipes. I created products from soaps to baby massage oils to spray mists that the kids think are for chasing monsters (of course, I really developed those blends to help them relax).

Make no mistake about it. Today's kids need to relax and feel less anxious. Stress is a health threat on par with chemical toxins. We need to reduce both surpluses in our lives, and especially in the lives of our children.

Research using the Rahe-Holmes scale of life-changing events (such as divorce, having kids, losing a job, death of a loved one, getting sued) shows stress has increased 45 percent in the last three decades. Moreover, a landmark study by the Families and Work Institute in New York shows the thing children would most like to change about their lives is, "having their parents less stressed and less tired." Seems like we all need some of *Earth Tribe Monster Mist* and other essential oils!

Researchers at the University of Wisconsin's Health Emotions Re-

Earth Healing (continued)

The instructions for use appeared almost too easy after so many months of visiting medical specialists: Place a cotton ball soaked in eight to ten drops of the *Sweet Dreams* blend under B.J.'s pillow, then wait for results.

Yet by the second morning, B.J. was feeling refreshed—and calm. He told his mother he simply felt peaceful with no urge to flail in his bed. The pillowcase cotton ball "smelled like a campfire" to B.J. He felt like his life was just beginning, grounded in a new sense of tranquillity and solidness. Within weeks, he had convinced many of his high school football teammates to use essential oils as a way to relax and energize before big games!

search Institute report that parents say their schedules are so overladen that they have less reserve to calm and soothe kids. A University of Michigan study of 2,394 U.S. families showed that nearly half of parents said they did not feel they had enough time for an adequate number of daily activities with their kids, such as reading together, talking, playing games, helping with homework, preparing food, or folding laundry.

Essential oils can't do your talking, reading, or playing for you, but they can certainly enhance your home environment and family energy levels. You can feel better, no matter how tight the schedule. The oils are safe for everyone, even babies. You can feel less stressed, which the top behavioral scientists and child development specialists are now saying is the single best strategy for improving a child's health. And, best of all, plant oils take virtually no time to use.

Here are twenty-one ideas for using essential oils with children, one for every year until they reach adulthood:

1. Use a clay pot diffuser with *Earth Tribe Euphoria* blend (main ingredients are orange and bergamot essential oils) in play areas to promote joy, happiness, and a sense of well-being. Use about twenty to thirty drops in the typical diffuser.
2. Put three to five drops of *Euphoria* in a bath for cranky kids.
3. For overactive kids, diffuse *Earth Tribe Calming* blend (lavender and chamomile essential oils) throughout any rooms frequently used. Or put five drops in a bath.
4. To settle down your child, try one to two drops of *Calming* blend on each pulse point.
5. The ideal bedtime essential oil is lavender. Diffuse in the bed-

room or place one to two drops on your child's pillow and/or favorite stuffed animal. Five to eight drops in the bath is another good idea.

6. Put several drops each of lavender and chamomile into two ounces of carrier oil (sweet almond, soybean, hazelnut, avocado, grapeseed, jojoba, olive) for a relaxing massage oil for baby or mom. Don't use mineral or baby oil because neither allows the essential oils to penetrate the skin and do their healing. Mineral oil is not good for a baby's skin. *Earth Tribe* makes a special *Mother and Baby Massage Oil*, which is gentle enough for infants, but still allows the essential oils to penetrate and nourish the skin.

7. Use several drops of lavender or chamomile essential oils in a carrier oil (or *Earth Tribe Lullabye Baby Rub*) to rub on an infant's stomach for colic.

8. Use *Earth Tribe Claire* spray (tea tree, eucalyptus, and lavender are active ingredients) as a general disinfectant. Spray on hands after wiping noses (and there's no tissue and/or sink available). Spray work surfaces and toys to kill germs. Spritz changing areas and bed linens. It's more effective than synthetic counterparts and 100 percent natural. It is one of our most popular products. Customers always reorder it, usually in multiple numbers to give to family and friends! Our *Claire* spray is named in honor of my mother-in-law, Claire Patton, who raised ten happy children in a healthy, predominantly chemical-free home.

9. Apply a few drops of lavender essential oil directly to cuts, scrapes, and burns to disinfect and promote healing. Lavender is good for preventing potential scars.

10. Use a compress with five to ten drops of lavender essential oil for sunburns or blisters. You can also put about fifty drops of lavender in *Earth Tribe Base Spray* for a cooling and calming skin spray.

11. For an all-purpose salve, try *Earth Tribe Comfort Cream*. Its active ingredients are the herb calendula, plus essential oils of lavender, tea tree, and chamomile. It is terrific for diaper rash, without the harsh chemicals, and equally good for cuts, scrapes, sunburn, dry and chapped skins, insect bites, and other rashes.

12. Tea tree essential oil is a marvel of nature. It can be applied directly to any cut, rash, scrape, or burn. Remember you don't need a lot.

Stretch Mark Alert

It might seem that I am pulling your leg or stretching the truth, but seriously, our *Earth Tribe Mother and Baby Massage Oil* will help prevent stretch marks from pregnancy. It has a gentle yet potent combination of lavender and chamomile. You can also try this homemade recipe: one ounce of carrier oil (avocado, sweet almond, jojoba) with seven drops of lavender essential oil and five drops of tangerine essential oil. I perfected the formula before having my twin boys, and you might hate me saying it, but I used the oil every day and didn't get a single stretch during nine months (plus post-delivery) of checking in the mirror.

As an added bonus, the oil serves as an all-purpose body moisturizer. You can use it daily any time you see stretch marks developing on the abdomen, breasts, hips or thighs.

Family of One (or More)

Every family needs a *sacred space* in the home, even if your family for the moment is me, myself, and I. The concept can be as simple or elaborate as you choose. I vote for simple. Pick a place in your home—even a nook or cranny—where silence is required whenever you are in that place. Keep a small bottle of lavender, eucalyptus, or another favorite essential oil in your sacred space (maybe a small table in the hallway is your pick of spots) and inhale it with at least three deep breaths every time you enter the area. Think of it as sort of a reduced speed zone in your life.

If you have room or the inclination or both, make your sacred space into a sitting area for meditation. Pillows on the floor can be an option, or maybe a set of chairs you and other family members found at a garage sale then refurbished. Aromatherapy candles and incense (make sure they contain pure essential oils) can enhance your sacred space. Your goal is to be silent and let your mind clear from the usual white noise of life.

13. For cold sores, for kids and adults alike, tea tree essential oil is very helpful. It is an antiviral oil. One to two drops on active cold sores will work wonders.

14. Tea tree essential oil can also address fungal infections, such as athlete's foot. Try ten drops in a footbath or apply it neat but sparingly to affected areas. If you don't have tea tree in the house, try lavender.

15. For gum infections and other cuts inside the mouth—don't miss this, all of you parents of inadvertent tongue-biters and inner-cheek chompers out there—a drop or two of tea tree essential oil will speed healing. If your child gets more than a few drops by mistake, flush the mouth with a glass or two of water.

16. For teething, place an infused warm compress with lavender and Roman chamomile on the appropriate cheek.

17. If your child is constipated, make a massage oil with seven to eight drops of geranium, rosemary, chamomile, or patchouli essential oils in two ounces of vegetable oil or any appropriate carrier oil. Give a daily massage at bedtime and make sure your child gets plenty of water and some fruit juice. Massage gently around the whole abdomen, moving clockwise to match the direction of the intestines.

18. For diarrhea, use a similar massage approach as described for constipation, but use a combination or single note of chamomile, geranium, sandalwood, and/or ginger. Another option is *Earth Tribe Tummy Tonic*. Also, it is best to avoid dairy products for about one week.

19. To protect against colds, flu, and fevers during winter months, place five drops each of lavender and eucalyptus or *Earth Tribe Breathe* in the child's bedroom humidifier each night. Another five drops of lavender in the bath helps fight infection, kill germs, and boost the immune system.

20. A fever can be reduced with a compress soaked in cool water with several drops of lavender.

Home Cooking

I was plenty busy in my kitchen during the early years of launching *Earth Tribe*. But the work paid off. Here is our line of *Tribe Kids* products. My husband and I use them every day with our own twin boys.

MONSTER MIST

This spray bottle (the perfect size for little hands to grasp) is filled with a *magical* formula that repels monsters and ghouls of all sorts when sprayed by a child throughout his or her room. The magical formula is actually a carefully chosen blend of essential oils clinically proven to calm, pacify, and comfort—while purifying and cleansing the air. It's 100 percent natural and nontoxic!

Directions: Have your child spray the bedroom or sleeping area with the *Monster Mist* to keep monsters at bay and to aid in calming and encouraging sleep.

Ingredients: pure spring water, essential oils of Bulgarian lavender, Roman chamomile, and sweet orange.

OWIE JUICE

A spray bottle with a blend of essential oils that disinfect, relieve pain, and promote the healing process (cell rejuvenation) for first-aid needs like cuts, scrapes, burns, insect bites, bruises, and sunburn. This formula is perfectly safe for topical applications and causes no side effects.

(continued)

Home Cooking *(continued)*

Directions: Spray on topically as needed.

Ingredients: pure spring water, powdered honey, aloe vera juice, essential oils of Bulgarian lavender, Australian tea tree, and Roman chamomile.

LULLABYE BABY RUB

This gentle baby oil is formulated with a blend of essential oils that help comfort, calm, and soothe babies. It works especially well when massaged on the tummy area for colic, and can also be used as a bath oil.

Directions: Gently massage on baby; for colicky babies, gently massage over tummy area. As a bath oil, place a small amount (1 tsp.) in baby's bath.

Ingredients: grapeseed oil, soybean oil, essential oils of Bulgarian lavender, Roman chamomile, and dill.

BABY BALM

A natural alternative to commercial diaper rash ointments that contain harsh synthetic chemicals. The perfect, natural solution for diaper rash, cradle cap, or any of the minor skin irritations that sometimes affect babies.

Directions: Apply topically to baby's skin as needed.

Ingredients: pure beeswax, soybean oil, calendula oil, aloe vera juice, and essential oils of Bulgarian lavender, Australian tea tree, and Roman chamomile.

HAPPY CHAP

This gentle, 100 percent natural lip balm is made with plant oils that have an aromatherapeutic effect of promoting joy and happiness. Very soothing and nourishing for dry, cracked lips. Comes in an easy-to-apply tube.

Directions: Apply topically on lips as needed.

Ingredients: pure beeswax, soybean oil, and essential oil of sweet orange.

PURE BOTANICAL BABY SHAMPOO & BATH GEL

This completely natural and gentle *no tears* antibacterial shampoo and bath gel is made without the harsh synthetic detergents found in most baby shampoos and bath gels. Excellent for babies' skin, including cradle cap.

Directions: Pour a small amount into your hands, then gently massage into a lather on child's hair, and rinse. As a bath gel, use in bath to cleanse body, or for a natural bubble bath, pour under faucet as you run the water.

Ingredients: purified water, aloe vera gel, coconut oil olefin, coconut oil betaine, avocado oil, lemon extract, essential oils of Australian tea tree and Bulgarian lavender and vitamins A, C, and E.

21. Use *Earth Tribe Breathe* blend (eucalyptus and fir balsam essential oils) as your family lookout during cold and flu season. Put five drops in each family member's humidifier. Put a couple of drops on everybody's pillows at bedtime. Put one or two drops in bath water or on a washcloth. You will cut down on colds, congestion, coughs, and sinus problems.

Chapter 9

Oils as Everyday Medicine

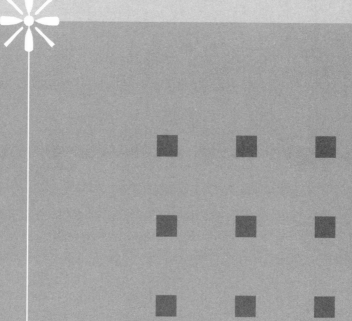

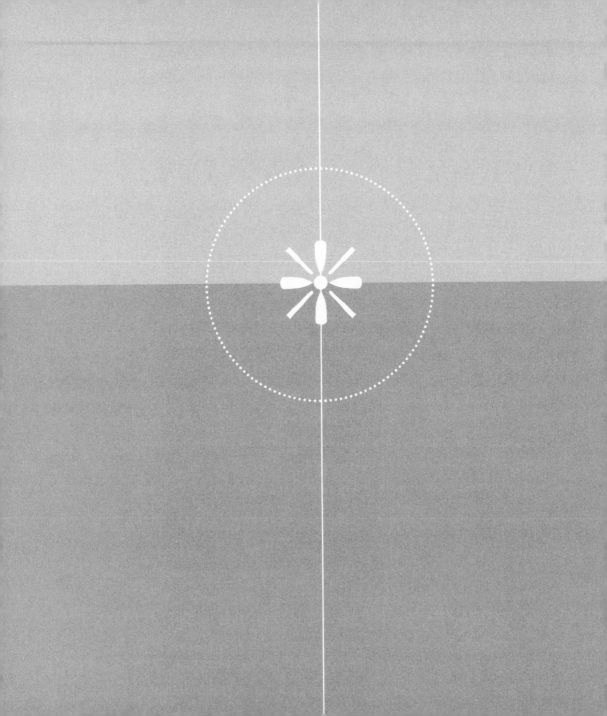

I've said it already, but the

message bears repeating. I am not a doctor. I don't pretend to be one, and I certainly don't want you to make any mistake on the subject.

In fact, a big reason why some people (especially some doctors) are skeptical about aromatherapy—and by association, essential oils—is because a few too many would-be aromatherapists play doctor and make false health claims. If you have a serious medical condition, see a physician. Get the best advice modern medicine can offer. Investigate alternative or complementary health therapies, such as herbal supplements and acupuncture. Then weigh all of your options and decide what treatment plan is best for you.

This doesn't mean I wouldn't recommend essential oils for anyone with serious or chronic problems. After all, I was once the twenty-one-year-old woman told by my doctors that my face, chest, and arms would be scarred for life. Essential oils do have incredible healing powers and life force, and they are always worth trying. They can produce miraculous results; however, just be sure to ask yourself whether you are relying on essential oils at the personal expense of ignoring a treatment option that could help more.

In any case, essential oils can change your life— and *healthstyle*—for the better. They shine most in what I call *everyday medicine* or the process of feeling as good as you can each day. We all want to feel better, no matter if we are relatively healthy or battling a chronic illness. Plant oils can replace harsh chemicals and medications in your medicine cabinet. They can unleash energy you didn't even know was inside you. They can help you feel more hopeful. They can dial down the artificial and turn up the natural.

This chapter covers how essential oils can be part of your own everyday medicine plan. I identify a number of conditions and circumstances that can be improved with certain plant oils, plus provide a first-aid kit of ideas that would suit Mother Nature herself. I have also included guidelines for pregnancy, and I promise you that I tested them all myself while I was carrying my twin boys!

There's more. Chances are you will like this concept: I think to be fully and naturally healthy, we need to take more baths and get more massages (both with essential oils, of course). Though it may sound like pampering—as if there were something wrong with that—there are sound, scientific reasons for my suggestions. Read on and you will see what I mean.

Address Stress

To start, I don't think it surprises any of us to discover that one of the hottest areas of scientific research involves the physical effects of stress. Researchers are making new discoveries practically every month about the damage chronic stress can do to the immune system or hormonal balance, especially among women. Other studies squarely point to too much stress as a risk factor for heart disease.

But there's hope for any of us with a stressful life, and wouldn't that be just about everyone, every day? For instance, research shows meditation can lower blood pressure in hypertensive individuals. Dr. Dean Ornish has used yoga as the core element for the stress-relief portion of his highly respected and documented program for reversing heart disease. Plus, a recent study reported one of the strongest predictors for better heart health among men aged thirty-five to fifty-nine is whether they take annual vacations. Those who do are 32 percent less likely to die prematurely from heart disease than guys who skip vacations.

I say essential oils can help you create situations that are like mini-vacations for the heart and other organs, such as the liver, that react adversely to too much stress. Research from such institutions as Harvard Medical School show even short breaks of ten to fifteen minutes each day can likely offset much of the potential damage. Using essential oils can become part therapy and part ritual that can be done in minutes or less.

For relief from stress and anxiety, use lavender or a blend of lavender and chamomile (the active ingredients in *Earth Tribe Calming* blend) with your favorite application method, including inhalation, compresses, massage, or baths. Place two drops of the same oils, or the *Earth Tribe Sweet Dreams* blend of lavender and marjoram, on your pillowcase at night for more restful sleep, which goes a long way to reducing the stress load on the body. For mild depression, try *Earth Tribe Balance* blend with rose and bergamot oils (bergamot alone is a good pick-me-up for down days).

Headaches are another symptoms of stress. Peppermint essential oil or the *Earth Tribe Head Peace* blend of basil and rosemary can neutralize tension headaches, plus help you ward off the triggers of the motherlode of headaches, the migraine. A drop or two rubbed into each temple or at the base of the skull is one strategy, though inhalation or a compress can work equally well. If you have only lavender at hand, it is an effective substitute.

More Everyday Oils for What Ails You

Here are some other common conditions and situations that can be improved with essential oils. Effective applications include inhalation, massage, compress, and bath/shower (and others as suggested below). Dilute pure essential oils in vegetable or nut oil (twenty drops essential oil in ¼ cup other oil), or in water for compresses. Note: Blends can often be more effective because of their synergistic nature. Remember to consult your health practitioner for any serious circumstances.

- Athlete's foot: Tea tree, eucalyptus, myrrh, lavender
- Black eye: Geranium, lavender (place two drops of each in a bowl of ice-cold water; soak a cotton ball in the liquid and place it over closed eye and surrounding affected area)

- Blemishes: Tea tree, lavender, eucalyptus (apply any of the three directly on blemishes), *Earth Tribe Tea Tree Face Wash* (See Chapter 10 for more skin care details.)
- Blisters: Geranium, lavender
- Chills: Geranium
- Colds: Eucalyptus, *Earth Tribe Breathe* blend (eucalyptus, fir), *Earth Tribe Cold and Flu Rub*
- Cold sores/canker sores: Tea tree (swab directly onto infected area three to four times daily). Also lavender on canker sores
- Constipation: Peppermint, thyme (never apply pure thyme essential oil directly to skin, and never swallow it)
- Cramps: Peppermint
- Diarrhea/gas: Ginger, lavender, chamomile, peppermint, *Earth Tribe Tummy Tonic* (gently massage over abdomen area)
- Dry, flaky skin: Geranium, lavender, melissa, *Earth Tribe Herbal Comfort Cream*
- Earaches: Tea tree, lavender, *Earth Tribe Calming* blend (lavender, chamomile) (place a few drops of selected oil in 1 tsp. warm olive oil; soak small piece of cotton in this mixture and place just inside the ear)
- Fatigue: Peppermint, geranium, black pepper
- Fevers: Eucalyptus, peppermint, lavender (use with a compress)
- Fluid retention: Grapefruit, lemon, juniper, rosemary, cypress, *Earth Tribe Slim-u-lite Massage Oil*
- Hay fever: Chamomile, eucalyptus

- Head lice: Tea tree, rosemary
- Heat exposure: Eucalyptus, peppermint, lavender
- Hemorrhoids: Patchouli, myrrh, cypress (make blend with five drops myrrh, two drops cypress, and one drop patchouli; place two drops on washcloth soaked in warm water; apply to affected area for a few minutes twice daily)
- Herpes: Tea tree, bergamot, geranium
- Gum infections: Tea tree (mix four drops with one tsp. of vegetable oil for swabbing on gums or place two drops of oil on swab and rub gently over affected area); peppermint, lavender (two drops of each in glass of water for a mouthwash)
- Indigestion/heartburn: Peppermint, ginger, *Earth Tribe Tummy Tonic* (blend of the two)
- Infections: Lavender, tea tree, chamomile, thyme
- Itching: Eucalyptus, peppermint
- Jet lag: Lavender, eucalyptus, geranium, lemongrass, grapefruit
- Muscle aches/stiffness/soreness: Peppermint, lavender, eucalyptus, chamomile, *Earth Tribe Muscle Soothe* blend (sweet birch, peppermint), *Earth Tribe Cooling Cream*
- Premenstrual syndrome: Clary sage, sweet fennel, geranium, chamomile, lavender, *Earth Tribe Even Tides* (clary sage, sweet fennel)
- Prickly heat: Geranium, chamomile, eucalyptus, lavender
- Rashes: Lavender, chamomile, eucalyptus
- Repetitive stress injury relief: Lavender, rosemary, marjoram

- Shaving cuts: Lavender (apply directly to razor to avoid nicks)
- Sleep problems/insomnia: Lavender, chamomile, *Earth Tribe Sweet Dreams* (lavender, marjoram; place four drops on your pillowcase)
- Sore throat: Tea tree, sandalwood (dilute three drops each in ¼ cup water for gargle; add a couple pinches of salt)
- Sprains/strains: Ginger, lavender, chamomile, *Earth Tribe Muscle Soothe*
- Sties: Lavender (one drop on cotton ball, rub on cheekbone under the sty, keeping eye closed); tea tree (four drops in bowl of purified water; soak cotton ball in this mixture and place over closed eyelid three times daily). Do *not* place essential oils directly into the eye.
- Sunburn: Lavender, peppermint, eucalyptus, chamomile
- Swelling/inflammation: Eucalyptus, lavender
- Toothache: Tea tree, clove (mix four drops total with one tsp. of vegetable oil for swabbing on gums or place two drops on swab and rub gently over affected tooth)
- Travel sickness: Ginger, peppermint, *Earth Tribe Tummy Tonic*
- Vomiting: Peppermint, ginger, lavender
- Warts: Tea tree (mix twelve drops in one ounce castor oil, apply several times daily with sterile dropper or applicator)
- Windburn: Lavender, eucalyptus, chamomile

First-Aid Kit

Here are some essential oils solutions when you have minor emergencies on your hands that seem big enough at the time.

- Bruises/bumps: Essential oils of lavender and geranium, two or three drops directly on area of bruise, or in a cold compress.
- Burns: Essential oil of lavender topically over the burn, also in cold compress. Then apply *Earth Tribe Herbal Comfort Cream* as needed.
- Cuts, scrapes, and wounds: For cleaning wounds, use ten drops of lavender in one cup of water (purified if possible) and pour over wound. Or use compress soaked in the water and lavender.
- Insect bites and stings: Apply tea tree and lavender to the bite. Also try geranium essential oil right on the bite. Treat painful stings, after removing the stinger, with a paste of lavender, tea tree, onion juice, cider vinegar, and baking soda.
- Nosebleeds: Soak a cotton ball in *Earth Tribe Plant Essence Skin Tonic* and plug the nose with it.

Pregnancy Pause

There has been debate about whether essential oils are appropriate during pregnancy. The controversy is basically about whether certain oils trigger spontaneous abortion or undesired uterine contractions. It sounds scary—especially during the early months of pregnancy—but certain oils have been deemed by more than a few researchers as safe for women carrying a baby. Consult your health practitioner if you have any doubts or a history of miscarriage (you might find midwives are generally more informed about oil use than are physicians). Here is the safe oils list, which comprises oils suitable for inhalation ONLY.

Safe Oils
Bergamot
Chamomile
Geranium
Lavender
Lemon
Neroli
Orange
Patchouli
Sandalwood

The idea is to choose more gentle oils that can still be effective for such discomforts as morning sickness, constipation, leg cramps, and overall fatigue. Before we talk about specific recipes, here are oils to AVOID during pregnancy. They are typically useful, but can overwhelm a woman and her baby in the delicate months of child-bearing:

Oils to Avoid
Angelica
Basil

- Black pepper
- Camphor
- Cedarwood
- Cinnamon
- Citronella
- Clary sage
- Clove
- Cumin
- Eucalyptus
- Fennel
- Hyssop
- Juniper
- Peppermint
- Rose
- Rosemary
- Sage
- Thyme

As in every case, respect the potency of essential oils. You should never ingest an essential oil without the supervision of a qualified health practitioner and aromatherapist, and doubly so when you are pregnant. Some women and practitioners prefer to avoid essential oils during the first trimester. During pregnancy, it is better to use plant oils in diluted amounts, such as seven drops of lavender and chamomile per ounce of carrier oil in the *Earth Tribe Mother and Baby Massage Oil*. Always keep in mind, less is more with plant oils.

My own pregnancy experience was greatly enhanced with the more gentle essential oils, which I prefer to drugs and other synthetic chemicals. Here are some of my favorite recipes for childbearing:

- Nausea/morning sickness: A woman's sense of smell is heightened during pregnancy. Some formerly pleasant aromas might now make her sick. Using a diffuser can help. Add one drop of lavender essential oil and three of lemon essential oil for morning sickness. To offset nausea, use a cool compress with two drops of lavender.

Coming Up Roses

Rose essential oil can help couples with fertility problems. Some aromatherapists recommend warm baths with four to ten drops of rose oil for men who want to maximize their sperm counts. A rose oil–infused massage oil (four to seven drops of rose oil per ounce of carrier) is good (and fun!) for couples massage.

Several essential oils can enhance a woman's fertility and help minimize the effects of stress. Make a massage oil with three drops of rose, four drops of geranium, three drops of clary sage, two drops of ylang ylang, and two drops of bergamot in two ounces of your favorite carrier oil. Use it for a nightly abdominal massage before bed. Gently rub the entire pelvic region in small, clockwise strokes. Use this only during the two weeks from menstruation to mid-cycle. Discontinue if you are or think you may be pregnant.

- Varicose veins: Elevate your legs when possible and use alternating warm and cold compresses with a couple of drops of lavender, lemon, or geranium.

- Edema (fluid retention around the feet and ankles): A tepid-to-cool foot bath with three drops of lemon, geranium, or lavender can help.

- Hemorrhoids: One of the less fun items on the pregnancy checklist. Get relief with a cool sitz bath containing six drops of lavender essential oil.

- Sleep problems: Nothing is any more important for an expecting mother than getting enough rest. I recommend sprinkling neroli, sandalwood, or chamomile oils around your bed, with a drop on the pillow. You can also take a soothing warm bath (again, not too hot) before bed. Add six drops of neroli for a peaceful night.

- Stretch marks: *Earth Tribe Mother and Baby Massage Oil* will help prevent stretch marks from pregnancy. It has a gentle yet potent combination of lavender and chamomile. You can also try this homemade recipe: one ounce of carrier oil (avocado, sweet almond, jojoba) with seven drops of lavender and five drops of chamomile. I used the formula while carrying my twin boys and never had a single mark. Use it daily any time you see stretch marks developing on the abdomen, breasts, hips, or thighs.

- Overall fatigue: Combine three drops of grapefruit and three drops of lavender in your bath or add six drops each to two tablespoons of carrier oil for a body rub.

As for labor and delivery, the research findings about essential oils are quite positive. A British study of 8,000 women—aromatherapy is a widely accepted practice in England—showed plant oils can significantly reduce anxiety and pain associated with childbirth. Less than 1 percent of women who used essential oils during labor needed painkiller drugs, compared to a national average of 30 percent. Close to 90 percent of the women said essential oils were moderately to extremely effective at reducing feelings of fear and anxiety.

Other studies, including some published by nursing researchers, confirm similar benefits of using essential oils during delivery. Here are some ways women find comfort: Lavender foot baths to stimulate circulation and relieve pain, clary sage massages to calm the nervous system and encourage breathing, and rose compresses to help soften ligaments and allow the pelvic bones to expand. Beware: Some oils, such as rose or clary sage, can be beneficial during delivery but still have their contraindications during the pregnancy. For more information about aromatherapist practitioners who can help with childbirth issues, contact the National Association for Holistic Aromatherapy at 888-275-6242 or check out www.naha.org.

Bath Time

It's cheap. It's easy. It's close by. Your bathtub could be your secret weapon in upgrading your healthstyle—and downsizing your stress levels. On the other hand, yeah, the one on the shower nozzle, the bathtub might just be the most overlooked place in your home. People tend to take the fast track these days, even in the bathroom.

While baths may be undervalued by most Americans, researchers in England have found that baths about sixty to ninety minutes before bedtime will increase the deeper stage-four and slow-wave sleep times during a night. In follow-up studies, our country's National Sleep Foundation has confirmed research that a fifteen-minute hot bath ninety minutes before bed is associated with falling asleep faster. Although the bath itself might raise body temperature, it then lowers the body's thermostat in the next hour and a half for optimal sleep temperature.

A recent study published in none other than the prestigious *New England Journal of Medicine* showed that soaking in a hot tub can reduce the need for insulin medication among patients with Type 2 or adult-onset

Checking the Temperature

Hydrotherapy is a required subject at the country's top massage schools. It reviews the ancient healing art of *taking the waters* for your health. While a hot springs spa might be the ideal place to tap into the health benefits of bathing, your own tub is a worthy alternative. Just be sure to not overdo it with the hot side of the faucet. A warm bath between 95 to 100 degrees is ideal for most people. A bath hotter than 100 degrees may cause problems for anyone with heart or circulation conditions, but it may provide relief for chronic pain. Anything over 104 degrees will be unbearable to most of us, though the Japanese bathe at temperatures closer to 110. You can use a cooking thermometer to help you develop an instinctive feeling for temperatures that best suit you.

diabetes. Researchers aren't sure exactly what produced the results, though one can speculate on the stress relief provided by taking a hot bath each day.

But America has too often drip-dried the notion of taking a bath, which needs to be at least fifteen minutes long—a half hour is optimal—for full therapeutic benefits (a fast hot bath can actually dehydrate you). In contrast, Moslems consider relaxed bathing a way to enlightenment. The Japanese use bathing as a means of maintaining balance with the forces of nature.

You can do your own nature balancing with baths, whether you can find time daily or make it a weekly ritual. Adding eight to ten drops of your favorite essential oil can transform a bath into a present-day form of the ancient art of hydrotherapy. Make sure to add the oil while the water is running so the bath is most effective. My recommendations include:

- To relax, use *Earth Tribe Calming* blend (it features lavender and chamomile essential oils).
- To revive, use *Earth Tribe Energize* blend (key ingredients are juniper and peppermint).
- For colds and flu, use three drops of lavender and three drops of tea tree oil.
- For children, try five to seven drops of lavender or the *Earth Tribe Calming* blend to calm, kill germs, and boost the immune system.
- For babies (newborn to two years old), use three to five drops of lavender or *Calming* blend.

- For a sensuous bath, try sandalwood, rose, ylang ylang, patchouli, neroli, jasmine, or *Earth Tribe Night Fire*.
- To soothe dry or flaking skin, opt for chamomile, lavender, patchouli, or sandalwood.
- Oils you should avoid in the bath include basil, oregano, thyme, nutmeg, cinnamon, clove, black pepper, bay, peppermint, and rosemary.

Getting in Touch

More and more doctors are recommending massage therapy as part of treatment. And the better news is, insurance companies are covering it more often, partly because there is research to support the protocol.

For example, a series of studies at the University of Miami Medical School showed that a thirty-minute neck-and-back massage reduces depression in subjects who were either trauma victims or touch-starved from lack of physical contact with others.

Other research shows massage therapy can alleviate chronic pain, inflammation, nausea, and epilepsy. You can expect more research in the years ahead. The National Center for Complementary and Alternative Medicine is funding even more studies.

The best-known style of massage therapy is the Swedish or Esalen technique, which is a gentle friction massage with long, flowing strokes. A second option is the shiatsu, based on the Japanese system in which critical pressure points are identified and released by pressing down with the thumbs or butt of the hand. Both styles are conducive to using essential oils.

A typical massage oil is about ten to fifteen drops of pure essential oil to two ounces of carrier oil. For example, six drops of sandalwood and three drops each of neroli and clary sage in the carrier is a good mix for stress relief. Or you can add six drops of lavender plus three drops each of chamomile and neroli for a sleep-promoting massage. Four drops of bergamot with two drops of geranium and one drop of melissa can lift your spirits.

If you see a massage therapist, you can bring along your own essential oils to add to the carrier oil he or she already uses. You might consider three drops each of grapefruit, geranium, and juniper to ward off cellulite or five drops of lavender plus two drops each of frankincense and rosemary for general aches and pains.

Earth Tribe has developed an entire product line of massage oils and aromatherapy rubs to save you the trouble of mixing and blending. Following are some possibilities.

Massage Oils

- *Mother and Baby Massage Oil*

  The gentle healing properties of lavender and chamomile combine to create a soothing all-over body moisturizer. Use throughout your pregnancy to keep skin smooth and soft and to help in preventing stretch marks. Keep this blend on hand post-delivery as it also makes a gentle, calming massage for the new baby. Active ingredients: lavender, chamomile.

Earth Healing

Michelle Kluck

Massage therapy keeps gaining more supporters in the medical community for its healing properties. It is no longer simply a luxury item on one's health checklist.

But Los Angeles–based massage therapist Michelle Kluck's clients already know that. Several celebrities have sought her healing touch for its energizing effects and to counter the high demands of their grueling schedules. Michelle has tried *Earth Tribe* essential oils and other products with Salma Hayek, Ashley Judd, and Peter Gabriel, among others. They loved the oils—and took them home, too!

"I love Mary Lee's whole product line," Michelle told my coauthor, Bob, during an interview. "I can tell the difference in quality between her oils and inferior ones on the market, and so can my clients."

Michelle is also a certified infant massage therapist who teaches regularly at southern

(continued)

- *Slim-u-lite Massage Oil*

  Quickly becoming a favorite, this blend is formulated with four essential plant oils that aid the body in breaking down stubborn fatty deposits and getting rid of excess water; it leaves the skin silky soft. Active ingredients: cypress, juniper, grapefruit, fennel.

- *Muscle Soothe Massage Oil*

  Relax and relieve discomfort in sore, tired muscles before or after strenuous activity. A great all-over body massage for the active. Active ingredients: peppermint, sweet birch, Roman chamomile, marjoram.

- *Calming Body Oil*

  A bestseller with massage therapists and

parents, this relaxing massage oil is the perfect rubdown for overworked, over-stressed adults; a terrific rub for calming little ones! Active ingredients: lavender, sandalwood, tangerine.

- *Night Fire Body Oil*

A highly sensual massage, bath, or body oil, this provocative formulation utilizes nature's most effective aphrodisiacs to help set the mood. Active ingredients: lavender, sandalwood, patchouli, clove, ylang ylang.

Earth Healing (continued)

California sites. She has made a popular video on baby massage (Living Arts) and uses only *Earth Tribe* children's products for her classes and video.

"Moms and dads love *Earth Tribe* products," says Michelle, whose new book *Hands on Feet* just came out from Running Press. "I give a kit to every new parent among my clients and students.

"I truly admire Mary Lee's message about getting chemicals out of our lives. Her oils are the right answer for anyone who wants to lead a more natural life. She lives what she believes."

- *Rejuvenator Massage Oil*

A unique blend of essential oils helps to improve circulation, while supporting the elimination of toxins in joints and tissues. Amazingly soothing and rejuvenating to tired and swollen feet and legs as well as other areas of the body. Active ingredients: cypress, peppermint, marjoram.

- *Volupte Body Oil*

    This luxurious body oil has been created with rare and precious pure essential oils that pamper your body and soul. Delight in the sensuous and pleasurable feelings of this blend. Active ingredients: vanilla, sandalwood, jasmine, rose.

Aromatherapy Rubs

- *Cold and Flu Rub*

    Utilizing nature's most potent ingredients, this traditional remedy rub helps to fortify the body while releasing toxins and easing the discomforts of cold and flu. It serves as triple threat of antibacterial, antiviral, and antifungal. Apply topically; for children and adults. Active ingredients: lavender, tea tree, manuka, eucalyptus.

- *PMS Relief Rub*

    This skillfully crafted formula, when applied over the lower abdomen and lower back, helps to relieve pain and discomfort associated with premenstrual syndrome. The balancing scent also lifts the spirits. Active ingredients: peppermint, marjoram, clary sage, geranium, chamomile.

Chapter 10

Rethinking Skin and Beauty Care

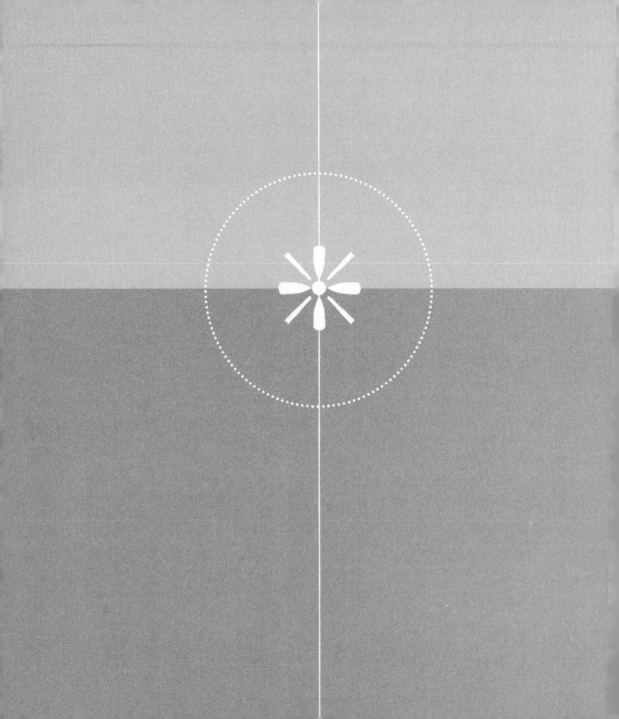

Picture dawn in a remote village in the highlands of Bulgaria. A small group of pickers are leaving a purple mist-covered field, their baskets overflowing with lavender flower tops. They begin to drift back to the "still house" to place the morning's harvest into the hands of the master distiller. Here the lavender flower tops are carefully examined and sorted by skilled hands before being put into the low-pressure, low-temperature still to extract the precious essential oil.

This is just the beginning of a unique and ancient process that will ultimately lead to one of our *Earth Tribe* beauty products. And this is why so many *Earth Tribe* customers say they can feel the vibrant energy when they use our products, and why skin care products from big, expensive department store brands seem lifeless in comparison.

I have three basic beliefs about skin and beauty care. It is important that you understand my perspective, even if you don't agree—at least not yet! Here's what I believe, in order from easiest to hardest to accept:

- It is relatively easy to agree with me that too many American women put too many synthetic chemicals on their faces, hair, hands, breasts, legs, you name it. Some government experts have estimated up to 200 chemicals a day! Not enough of U.S. women know that the skin is the body's largest organ and, even if they do know, they aren't checking the ingredients of their favorite skin creams, lipsticks, or makeup very closely—if at all. While everybody wants to look beautiful, it shouldn't come at any price. Our bodies, especially our skin, need a respite from harsh chemicals.

- The second belief might take more of a leap of faith, or imagination, on your part. But here goes: I believe essential oils have a life force that can be transferred to, say, the skin, when applied. Plant energy becomes your energy. Okay, woo woo, you're thinking, and what about the fact that plants are *killed* to make the oils? Typically, the plant is harvested for its flowers or leaves or even stems but it grows back the next season. The harvested part of the plant is immediately processed to lock in maximum freshness and life force. As for the woo woo, I simply have seen too many examples—with my own facial burns, healing stories of clients (including my great

Label Able

So-called natural beauty products aren't always as advertised. Manufacturers might indeed use natural ingredients but in tiny amounts compared to the artificial substances used. You can check out any product's claim by looking at the label. By federal law, ingredients are listed in descending order, starting with the greatest amount in the product. A moisturizer with a featured ingredient close to the beginning of the list, for example, would have more of that ingredient than any other ingredient. A featured ingredient listed close to the end suggests that not much of that ingredient is present.

And while you are at it, you might note that a product labeled as, say, lemon or rosemary doesn't contain a single drop of essential oil.

friend Gina Belafonte profiled in this chapter), and research studies—to believe there isn't real life force energy at work.

• You've heard my third belief before, or at least something like it: Beauty is not only in the eye of the beholder but also inside the heart and soul of each one of us. There's an old saying that "contentment is the best cosmetic for a woman's face." I agree, and suggest we are all happier when there are fewer chemicals and more natural substances in our lives. Think of it this way: Being positive about yourself equates to natural ingredients and self-doubt to harsh chemicals. Add the former, let go of the latter. The Natural Beauty portion of my Healthy Living plan is aimed squarely at accomplishing a new balance in your life with essential oils.

But don't just take my perspective for it. A short of history of beauty (without the textbook!) can help explain why essential oils are the missing ingredient in your personal care routine. We can all learn from the past to thrive in the future.

For thousands of years women all over the world, from all tribes and all cultures, have used plants to preserve their youthful looks, to soften their skin, to embellish, to cleanse, to tone, and to perfume themselves. The expertise of using plants for body and skin care was handed down from generation to generation, from mothers to daughters. There was nothing magical or mystical about it; specific plants were used for specific purposes because they worked. Simple as that. Natural as that.

Here are some historical examples of oils that were popular for skin and beauty care then and now:

- *Geranium*

  Native Americans have used the geranium plant as a cure-all for everything from toothaches to ulcers. Since ancient times, geranium has been used to balance female hormones and ease anxiety. But it has been most widely used to treat skin problems, due to its healing abilities. According to folklore, geranium was planted outside and around the home to protect it from evil spirits. That is a tradition that has remained, and it is why geraniums are the most common plants on doorsteps today. It is ideal for balancing your skin, but also for soaking up oily spots and even temporarily tightening mature skin.

- *Juniper*

   In ancient Egypt, juniper was one of the major ingredients used in the embalming process (imagine what it can do for our bodies!). It was also massaged onto the body or used in baths. Juniper oil was used as an effective diuretic to help control weight. In China and Tibet, Juniper was used to prevent infectious disease and to ward off evil spirits.

- *Lavender*

   To ward off the epidemics that occasionally went through their cities, the ancient Greeks, Romans, and Persians all burned lavender-flower tops. Lavender tales tell of its magical ability to promote states of blissful love and sensuality. Some Native American tribes have used lavender for centuries to heal burns, cuts, and scrapes.

- *Patchouli*

   This essential oil played an important role in the traditional medical systems of China, India, Japan, and Malaysia, as a general body tonic, a potent aphrodisiac, and an antidepressant. When the British stopped importing fabrics from India, and started manufacturing them themselves, the British women would not buy the fabric because it was missing the scent of patchouli. That's what I call a fashion statement!

- *Rose*

The ultimate symbol of love, the rose is found on the walls of Egyptian tombs dating back as far as 500 B.C. In ancient mythology the rose is linked and represented by the goddesses of love, Aphrodite and Venus. These days, aromatherapists revere it for moisturizing sensitive, dry, itchy, or inflamed skin, and for alleviating grief and anger.

There is a popular legend that the essential oil of rose was discovered at a Persian wedding. The royal affair was held at a palace surrounded by a canal. Roses and rose petals were thrown into the water as part of the celebration over a few days, and at the end of the festivities, a layer of essential oil was visible on top of the water in the canal. Smart merchants collected the rose oil in vessels, and a new trade was born.

- *Rosemary*

Rosemary has been honored and utilized in many ancient traditions. In Latin, rosemary translates to "dew of the sea," referring to the areas where it grows and flourishes. Greek philosophers wore garlands of rosemary to help their memories and sharpen their minds, while Queen Elizabeth of Hungary used rosemary and lavender in her famous facial potion still called Hungary Water. Though it might be part fable and part fact, the special liquid apparently made the

Queen so radiant and young-looking that the king of Poland proposed marriage when she was seventy-two.

Rosemary is for remembering, and is often placed on graves and at burial sites of loved ones. It is also a wonderful tonic for hair and scalp.

Somewhere between Queen Elizabeth and *Queen for a Day* we lost our connection to essential oils. By the middle of the twentieth century, most plant essences were being dismissed as old-fashioned. The petrochemical industry was blossoming, and big companies were convincing the public that the future of skin and body care was in the laboratory, where the new synthetic wonder creams were being made.

Discovering the ingredients of these creams is something of a wonder in itself! Glance at most any mass-produced cosmetics label and you will feel like you are in chemistry class rather than a department store. For instance, moisturizers and lotions might list propylene glycol, isopropyl myristate, and glycerin as active ingredients, plus artificial fragrances made from petroleum (yep, the same basic compound that goes into your car's gas tank).

You are what you eat, and what you put on your body and hair every day. Most American skin and beauty care products contain synthetic chemicals with emulsifiers, preservatives, disinfectants, sudsing agents, and sulfates. That's not much of a reflection upon us, and worse, the preservatives and disinfectants can impair or even eliminate the effectiveness of any botanical substance they may contain. These agents (formaldehyde, hexachlorophene, diazolidinyl urea, quarternium-15) are foreign substances that are known to damage the skin's flora and protective layer.

What's more—as if we really need more reasons to stop using harsh chemicals on our faces and bodies—many of the synthetic ingredients in face creams and cleansers can age the skin by reducing its water-absorbing capacities and decreasing the skin's elasticity. The wrinkles that result from this process? They're probably going to be treated with an antiaging cream that also contains harmful ingredients. The vicious cycle continues.

The skin is your body's first shield against environmental impurities, such as chemicals, pollutants, bacteria, and ultraviolet rays. It certainly doesn't help matters if your beauty products are adding to daily chemical exposure. My skin care program, detailed in this chapter, is simple but powerful in its dual purposes of nourishing your skin with essential oils and closing the (medicine cabinet) door on harsh synthetic chemicals.

It starts with the basics. What soap do you use in the shower? On your face? Many commercial soaps contain synthetic detergents and other chemicals that actually dry out and irritate the skin's outer layer or epidermis. They might contain mineral oil, which actually clogs pores and can be difficult to rinse out.

A true soap is made up solely of fats and an alkali. In the past, people made their own soap from animal fats and wood ashes. Still, today if a soap label doesn't specifically say it is vegetable-based—one popular combination is palm and coconut oils, but I prefer olive oil, especially from the Castile region of Spain—it is likely made from some form of animal fat. As for the ashes, manufacturers now use lye, which is the active ingredient in ashes.

Good news for us. More natural health companies are making and marketing good old-fashioned soap. But be careful about trusting the

See to It

For tired or puffy eyes, try this energizer. Fold two tissues into two-inch squares. Moisten tissues with cold water, then place in a small bowl filled with ice cubes for three minutes. Spritz the tissue pads with *Earth Tribe Plant Essence Skin Tonic* (active ingredients are lavender, witch hazel, cypress, juniper, and geranium essential oils). Place pads on eyes and leave on for two minutes, and then blink twenty times to get your blood circulating. Feel free to repeat daily if desired.

word natural in the label. Check the ingredients to make sure, including whether pure essential oils are actually used. Some soaps without special claims on cleansing or medicating don't have to list ingredients provided they use only forms of fat and alkali. I say honesty is the best and only policy. If a company doesn't want to tell me what's in its soap, then I don't need to give them my money.

Foaming agents in most popular bubble baths and shower gels also attack the skin flora, which makes the skin extremely dry and brittle. Many companies that include these agents in their products do so for two reasons: (1) they foam and clean quickly, and (2) they are readily available and cheap. It's also important to note that extensive animal testing was done with these agents in the 1960s, but because it was so long ago, most companies that use these substances also advertise that they are "cruelty free."

A spin through the U.S. Food and Drug Administration Web site re-

The science of skin care is simple: Skin can be treated successfully from the outside, because our skin absorbs as well as it excretes. This alone should make us rethink using beauty products that contain harsh synthetic chemicals. Our skin is already stretched to the limits by sunlight, wind, air pollution, chlorinated water, and poor nutrition. It makes good sense to not add to the body more synthetic chemicals in our beauty products.

When we use plant extracts on our skins we are using substances biologically compatible with our bodies, which they have no problem absorbing and assimilating. We have evolved with plants for thousands of years, and they can feed, tone, moisturize, stimulate, and revitalize far more effectively than any wonder chemical. Here is the *Earth Tribe* skin care program, which is based on a three-step daily program of cleansing, toning, and moisturizing the face:

CLEANSING

Twice daily, A.M. and P.M.

Cleansing in the morning is important to remove waste that your skin generates during the night. Before bed, you remove bacteria, oils, makeup, and other residues from the day.

I recommend *Earth Tribe Tea Tree Face Wash,* which unlike most liquid cleansers has no artificial detergents. Great for problem skin because of the natural antiseptic qualities of lavender and tea tree oil.

TONING

Twice daily, after cleansing.

I recommend *Earth Tribe Plant Essence Skin Tonic*. Each of its active ingredients makes a contribution without any drying and irritation to the skin. Cypress improves circulation, juniper decreases puffiness, extract of witch hazel tightens the pores, and lavender and tea tree essential oils have anti-inflammatory properties that are quite helpful to anyone with acne or oily skin.

Apply the toner with a cotton ball. A tip for guys: The toner makes an excellent aftershave, and the cypress helps stop bleeding from razor cuts.

MOISTURIZING

Moisturizing the skin is important because you establish a protective layer between your skin and everyday dirt, bacteria, and toxins. A moisturizer with essential oils helps nourish and soften the skin while protecting it. Plus, you can diminish fine lines on the face.

I recommend trying one of the *Earth Tribe Balancing Infusion* oils. Each one is formulated for a certain skin type, as outlined below. All of them contain the rare macadamia nut oil, which most closely represents the oils of our skin.

• *Balancing Infusion Number One*, with the cell-regenerating benefits of lavender and frankincense essential oils and the balancing effects of rose and geranium, is designed for dry/mature skin. Tip: If your skin is extremely dry, add two to three drops of sandalwood to the face oil when applying it to your face.

(continued)

Everyone, Every Day Skin Care (continued)

- *Balancing Infusion Number Two* is designed for normal/oily skin, with the antibacterial properties of tea tree and eucalyptus essential oils and the soothing effects of lavender.

- *Balancing Infusion Number Three* is for sensitive skin that has tendencies toward dryness. Its Roman chamomile and sandalwood essential oils quickly calm and restore the natural balance of the skin, while the lavender and evening primrose oils aid in cellular rejuvenation.

- *Balancing Infusion Number Four* is carefully crafted for problem skin, such as rosacea and blemished skin. This unique infusion contains healing helichrysum and a rare carbon dioxide extract of chamomile that work to quickly calm, clear, and balance the skin.

COMPRESS
Weekly.

In my skin care program, a compress helps deep clean the pores, improve circulation, and deep moisturize the skin. Simply soak a small towel in warm water infused with five to seven drops of essential oils. Then wring out the water, place the towel on your face, and luxuriate! Here are the best oils for your skin type:

- Oily skin: lavender, bergamot, geranium, patchouli, rose, rosemary, sandalwood, tea tree

- Normal skin: lavender, geranium, patchouli, rosemary, sandalwood, rose
- Mature skin: geranium, lavender, rose, rosemary, sandalwood
- Sensitive skin: rose, lavender, sandalwood, chamomile

EXFOLIATING THE BODY

Three to four times weekly.

Don't forget the skin beyond your face. You can look and feel better by paying more attention to all of your skin, especially trouble spots like the chest, back, knees, elbows, and feet. Exfoliating the body removes dead skin cells and gives the skin a smooth, silky appearance and feel.

I recommend *Earth Tribe*'s *Invigorating Mint Salt Glow* to jump-start your day, or revitalize tired, sore muscles. You can use it in the shower or bath to scrub the body. Some of our customers prefer *Earth Tribe*'s *Citrus Salt Glow* to refresh and rejuvenate. Both will pamper and detoxify your skin without causing any sensitivity or overdrying.

veals all sorts of potential problems with commonly used cosmetic products. Side effects can range from mild rashes to skin burns, from burning eyes to blindness.

Sure, cosmetics manufacturers might put some warnings about the consequences of misuse on their labels, and there are detailed directions for use. But most people figure that if the product is sold at stores it must be safe. Want an example? Detergent-based bubble bath products may irritate skin and the urinary tract through excessive use or prolonged exposure. The labeling instructs users to discontinue the product if rash, redness, or itching occur, to consult a physician if irritation persists, and to keep out of reach of children. These adverse reactions reportedly occur mostly with prolonged soaks. But I'm guessing very few people—adults or kids—equate bubble baths with anything potentially harmful.

Despite all of this chemical warfare—or is it *war paint?*—from multinational beauty products corporations, I am happy to report a change for the better. At least from every seminar I lead about essential oils,

Female Fact

The breast area needs special care. European women have long sworn by the "phyto-hormone" rich plant essences (geranium, rose, lavender, clary sage, and fennel) contained in our *Earth Tribe Cleavage Oil*. Massage on breast area twice daily to help moisturize, improve circulation, and enhance the skin's texture and tone.

Sensitive Subject

While everyone's skin is sensitive to any element that might damage it, some people feel it more in terms of dryness, reddening, inflammation, and rashes. Before trying any new skin care product, always do the wrist test. Place a dab or a few drops of the product on the back of one wrist. Rub it in with the other wrist. Wait a few hours to see if there is any adverse reaction.

every order, every new sales consultant that joins *Earth Tribe*, every talk show or media appearance I make, every friend who starts asking questions once she realizes what I do for a living. We as women instinctively know what is best for our bodies, and the dismissal of plants and essential oils has turned out to be relatively brief.

As we step comfortably into the new millennium—and actually grow accustomed to starting the year part of a date with the number "2"—the notion of using high-tech synthetic products on our faces and bodies is now what seems outdated and unhealthy. Most of the research for the plant ingredients that we do use today has been done for us over thousands of years, by countless women, and even the most brilliant findings cannot be patented (which is why big companies always alter the plant ingredient to get a patent).

Studies in Europe have found that the skin can only absorb 10 percent of most synthetic creams. This is mostly due to the large molecules of the active substances that cannot penetrate the upper layer of the skin.

It should tell you all you need to know that many soaps and body cleansers on the market today feature synthetic detergent products as active ingredients. How did we go from grandma's homemade recipes to FDA hearings and warnings about certain products we use to wash our faces and children's bodies?

The detergent cleansers are popular because they make suds easily in water and don't leave a gummy ring or deposit. Even the FDA recognizes that Americans can pay a price for such conveniences as not having to worry about a ring around the tub. Here is an excerpt from an FDA position paper on soaps:

"Soaps and synthetic detergent cleansing agents function in water in somewhat the same way; that is, they break down the resistance barrier between the water and the dirt, grime, oil, or other material, allowing it to be wetted and washed away. Soap works well in soft water, but in hard water, which contains a relatively high amount of calcium in solution, the calcium and soap react to form a gummy material called soap scum, which includes dirt and other matter. This gummy stuff is what forms the familiar ring in the bathtub.

"The increasing number of synthetic detergent bars on the market is due largely to their more efficient functioning in water, regardless of hardness, and because they don't form gummy deposits as does soap.

"There are many types of synthetic detergents, ranging from strong to mild; usually the milder types are used for personal cleansing. Some of the harsher detergents are capable of causing eye irritation or injury and manufacturers normally avoid using these in personal bathing bars. There are consumers who

may experience irritation or allergic skin reactions from some synthetic detergents. Some consumers also may be allergic to fragrances, colors, or other
substances added to either soaps or synthetic detergent bars."

So, in most cases, 90 percent of the cream or lotion sits on the face, un-
able to nourish the skin. It is difficult and costly to produce cosmetic and
beauty products that are to last for months or even years on retail shelves
without preservatives.

In contrast to synthetic, mass-produced personal care products, essential oils have small enough molecules to penetrate the skin's layers to
produce a rejuvenating effect. The plant oils get through to lower layers
of skin, which allows moisturizing and recovery from damage caused by
sun, burns, or wrinkling. Moreover, deeper penetration means the essential oils can reduce puffiness or inflammation and help regulate oily
and dry skin.

You gain by subtracting out the harsh chemicals of mass-produced lo-

Earth Healing

Gina Belafonte

Gina Belafonte was a client of *Earth Tribe* for almost two years when she realized she had been using many of the products but nothing for her face. That was unusual and understandable at the same time, because she has a skin condition called rosacea. It is an acne-like facial condition that causes redness on the cheeks, nose, chin, or forehead. If not treated, the redness becomes ruddier and more permanent.

"I had been using a product, MetroGel, recommended by my dermatologist," says Gina. "I was told it was a bit toxic and shouldn't be used while pregnant. Now I thought to myself, If I shouldn't use it when I'm pregnant, why should I really use it at all?"

So Gina asked me if there was any existing product or something I could develop. As it turned out, the MetroGel wasn't helping much anyway.

After doing some research about rosacea, I developed an essential-oil blend that Gina soon started calling a "magic brew." It is now the *Earth Tribe Balancing Infusion No. 4,* a unique infusion that contains helichrysum and a rare carbon dioxide extract of chamomile that work to quickly calm, clear, and balance the skin.

Gina stopped using anything on her face for about a week. She got fast results.

"Presto, within hours, truthfully, my skin felt calmer and so soothed," says Gina. "I kept using it and within a week or so my skin had never looked better."

Gina was so impressed, she signed up to become an *Earth Tribe* consultant her-

(continued)

self. She introduced *Earth Tribe* essential oils and products to her sister, actress, model, and TV host Shari Belafonte, and her famous father, Harry Belafonte.

"We all used the products for cleaning and personal care," says Gina. "My sister really appreciates the peppermint oil for preventing ants. The idea is the scent repels the ants—you can almost see them doing the backstroke to get away.

"I even got my mother to try tea tree oil for a rash on my four-year-old, Maria. She would traditionally use a cortisone-based cream, but tried the tea tree oil. Maria's rash cleared right up. My mother loved that."

Gina is a believer across the product line.

"I got rid of everything—shampoos, cleansers, soaps," says Gina. "Essential oils can do all of the jobs better."

I am grateful to Gina for her enthusiasm about *Earth Tribe* products, but even more excited that she has signed on to become the company's executive vice-president for the new *Earth Tribe* spa product line.

Gina's marketing work is already producing dividends. *Earth Tribe Citrus Salt Glow* is used for exfoliation on the hands and feet at la vie l'orange, a nail salon that Oprah Winfrey called one of her twenty-five favorite things, in a recent issue of *O Magazine*.

tions, creams, makeup, and other skin care products. Our *Earth Tribe* line contains no mineral oils (which sound natural enough but can damage the skin, especially on babies and young children), alcohols, synthetic preservatives, or dyes. The vegetable and nut oils we use as bases and carrier oils also have excellent skin care qualities, contain nutrients, and regulate moisture.

Of course, we feature the best nutrients you can *feed* your skin: essential plant oils. Essential oils naturally cleanse the skin of harmful bacteria that may cause blemishes; they help to improve the circulation in the skin, bringing more oxygen and nutrients to the skin; they stimulate cell rejuvenation, a key to younger-looking skin; and they relieve stress with their aromatherapeutic qualities. Remember what I said about contentment and beauty!

I can't say it enough and hope you come to agree with me: An important reason to use essential oils in skin and body care is to receive their vital energy force. The life within us can best be cared for and healed with living things. When the skin is being treated with plant oils, it is receiving the solar energy and life force of the plant. You will get physical results from essential oils—and there's nothing wrong with that—but the effect will go deeper to the core of your being. You will simply look better and feel better, more energized and rested and peaceful, especially about yourself. Now that's what I call a beautiful thing.

Chapter 11

Detoxing Your Beauty Routine

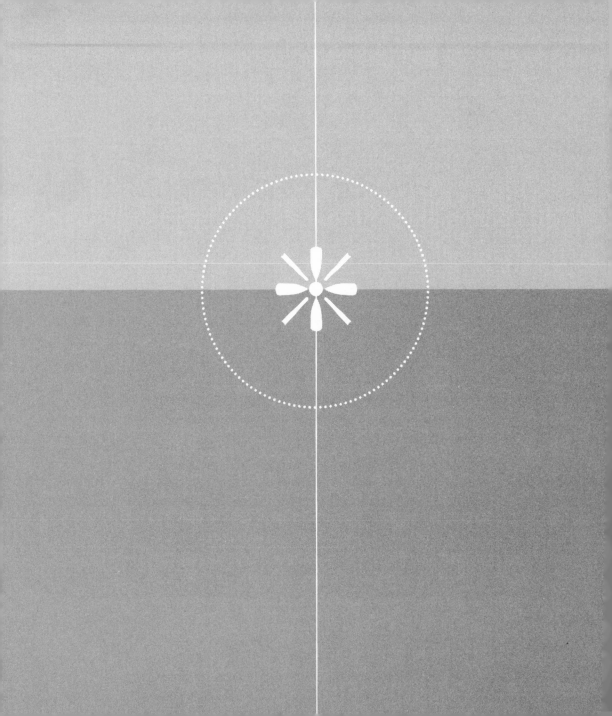

Let's face facts, beauty starts with

the skin. We just covered this important subject in Chapter 10. But, of course, beauty and personal care is more than skin deep. That's why we have talked about self-confidence and increasing your verve in earlier chapters. My coauthor, Bob, says there is nothing sexier than a woman who believes in herself, and who's to argue! Feeling good about yourself—and getting the chemicals out of your life is the best way to start—can transform you in the eyes of all those beholders out there.

What remains is a practical discussion about parts of the beauty regimen that occupy lots of our time but not always with best results. Ever heard of bad hair days? Essential oils can turn those around. The same goes for brittle nails, dull teeth, breast stretch marks, and cellulite.

The first step is realizing how many chemicals are "polluting" our personal care products. There are almost too many to count. Here are some common beauty issues and how you can close down the chemicals and open the possibilities:

Bad Hair Days (or Weeks or Months)

Consider shampoos, even ones claiming to be all-natural. Here we find strong alkaline soaps that are not beneficial to the skin, and the ever-present sodium lauryl sulfate, cocomide DEA, cocomide MEA, and TEA lauryl sulfate, all wetting agents that foam and clean. You get lots of suds with even just a dab. They clean so thoroughly, in fact, that the protective acid mantle and the skin's natural sebum are completely washed away. As a result, the scalp is off balance, and the hair that grows from it is damaged.

There is controversy about the safety of sodium lauryl sulfate, which even its supporters concede can cause eye irritation, skin rashes, and allergic reactions in some people. Others point out that it is a toxic chemical, not to be swallowed or inhaled in its raw form, that independent lab tests show may be harmful if simply absorbed through the skin.

Sodium lauryl sulfate is used for two primary reasons. It is cheap, and it foams up a mixture quite well. It thickens easily when mixed with salt, which is also cheap. Some companies have reacted to the buzz about sodium lauryl sulfate and substituted sodium laureth sulfate, which they deem as less abrasive or threatening. But I say no matter what side you take, we should know more about the potential health threats of sodium lauryl sulfate than we do. Let's prove beyond any doubt that these chem-

A Good Hair Night

About every week to ten days, make a date with yourself for a scalp massage using essential oils. You can make an appointment at a local spa, but here is a *home kit* checklist.

Oils: For dry hair and scalp, use sweet almond oil, just enough to drench hair but not leave it dripping, with ten to fifteen drops of chamomile, geranium, or rosemary essential oil premixed into it.

For oily hair and scalp, mix a blend of jojoba oil and ten to fifteen drops of juniper or lavender essential oil. Same thing, just enough to drench your hair but not have it drip. You can substitute tea tree or eucalyptus essential oils for the juniper to work on a dandruff problem.

How to massage: Apply oil to dry, unwashed hair. Start with the ends and move toward scalp. Always work the hair in a downward motion or direction of growth. Comb through and leave on hair for twenty minutes to overnight. Some people like to use a blow-dryer to spread the oils on the hair, but be sure not to use a hot setting.

icals won't hurt us or our children. Until then, why should we take our chances? Especially because sodium lauryl sulfate basically dries out and dulls your hair anyway. You get split ends and flyaway hairs. Even the plain old salt in the mixture can cause itching and even some hair loss.

Many beauty experts recommend not overshampooing your hair,

keeping it to about three times per week. What they mean, intended or not, is don't use so much sodium lauryl sulfate (or its DEA, MEA, or TEA cousins).

Essential oils can help solve your hair problems almost instantly. Dry hair is basically a matter of too little oil at the scalp line. Once a hair grows visible, it relies on oil from the scalp to coat it and keep it alive as long as possible. Shampooing with harsh chemicals just takes more oils away. Another problem: A dry scalp sheds skin too quickly, leaving immature follicle cells to handle the job of holding hair in place and providing oils. These cells aren't ready for the task, so your scalp becomes irritated and inflamed, feeling itchy or even painful.

To fix the problem, you can apply essential oil (diluted in olive oil) directly to the scalp with massage. It breaks up and lifts dirt, flaky skin, and other residues (some from artificial shampoos or *product buildup* as professionals call it) while not disturbing the helpful oils your scalp is producing. The essential oil and the massage itself also improve circulation to the scalp, which, being at the top of the head, is one of the most difficult places for the body to send blood.

What's more, replacing sodium lauryl sulfate with essential oils can *age-proof* your scalp. Follicles can age like any other part of our bodies, closing up and squeezing out hairs while not allowing new ones to grow. Cleaning out the scalp's pores and bringing more blood (and nutrients) to the area helps keep the follicles in good working order.

My solution to problem hair is *Earth Tribe Pure Botanical Shampoo* and *Earth Tribe Pure Botanical Conditioner.* Both products have no harsh chemicals and work wonders with essential oils of rosemary (great for all sorts of hair challenges), patchouli, lavender, and tea tree. It won't lather as much as a typical shampoo but you will notice the healthy difference in your hair.

You can also add the oils—especially rosemary for problem hair and the lavender/tea tree combination for dandruff—to your favorite natural shampoo. Just make sure it truly is natural!

Hair-Raising Consciousness

Here are the best essential oils for your hair, divided into dry and oily. Try adding five to ten drops of these oils to your favorite natural shampoo or using a few drops while you brush your hair briskly enough for coverage in the shower in a front-to-back, back-to-front motion. It helps treat the scalp and get the essential oils to the *nerve centers* of our hair, the follicles. You can also rub a few drops directly onto the scalp after washing, leaving it on for three to five minutes before rinsing.

For Normal Hair
Lavender
Lemon

For Dry Hair
Cedarwood
Chamomile
Geranium
Patchouli
Rosemary

For Oily Hair
Eucalyptus

Helichrysum

Juniper

Lavender

For Dandruff
Eucalyptus

Tea tree

For Hair Loss
Peppermint

Rosemary

Nailing It

No, there isn't an *Earth Tribe* nail polish. You are on your own there. But what essential oils can do is keep your nails strong and healthy—you may not want to use much polish to show them off! Anyone who works with essential oils, such as aromatherapists and massage therapists, will say that all that dipping of the hands in oils leads to beautiful nails that grow fast.

This is one part of your beauty regimen that can use a chemical over-haul. By all means, avoid nail builder products (elongators, extenders, hardeners, and enamels). They can irritate and inflame the nail bed, even cause infections, because of residues from chemicals called methacrylate monomers. Nail hardeners and enamels often contain formaldehyde and formaldehyde-releasing preservatives, which may cause allergic reactions in people sensitive to them and have been listed as a hazardous chemical by the Environmental Protection Agency.

Instead, here some simple but effective recipes for nail care. You will be amazed at the difference plant oils can make.

- *Nail strengthener blend*
  Two teaspoons grapeseed oil
  Five drops jojoba oil
  Three drops carrot essential oil
  Eight drops lemon essential oil
  Two drops rosemary essential oil

How to use: Make up a batch of this blend, then store it. Add the blend to one teaspoon of avocado or sweet almond oil. Massage well into the fingers and nails/toes and nails after a manicure/pedicure.

- *Cuticle softener blend*
  One teaspoon jojoba oil
  Five drops carrot essential oil
  Two drops eucalyptus essential oil
  Two drops peppermint essential oil

How to use: Massage the mixture well into cuticles. This should be the right amount for one session; you can double or triple the recipe for storage. But to maintain maximum potency, don't make too much at one time.

- *Fungus fighter*

  One teaspoon jojoba oil

  Five drops carrot essential oil

  Two drops lavender essential oil

  One drop oregano essential oil

  Two drops tea tree essential oil

How to use: If you've been diagnosed with a fungal infection, this blend can nurse your nails and cuticles back to health. Apply with clean swab tips.

- *Nail infection oil*

  Two tablespoons vegetable oil

  Ten drops tea tree essential oil

  Five drops eucalyptus essential oil

  Five drops patchouli essential oil

How to use: For general infections around the nail bed. Apply three times daily, massaging well.

Pointing the Finger

The following essential oils are good for strengthening nails:

Carrot

Cypress

Eucalyptus

Grapefruit

Lavender

Lemon

Rosemary

The following essential oils help fight nail infections:

Calendula

Eucalyptus

Lavender

Manuka

Myrrh

Oregano

Patchouli

Tea tree

Thyme

Eyes Have It

Eye makeup is a product monitored by the Food and Drug Administration's Office of Colors and Cosmetics. Serious injury is rare but the chemicals (especially preservatives) in mascara and eye shadow can cause irritation and allergic reactions in some women. Mascara wands can actually introduce microbacteria into the eye if you accidentally poke yourself (a good reason not to apply it while driving).

But even the safest use of makeup only covers up the bags or darkening, puffiness, crow's-feet, and other creased or sagging skin under and around the eye. The skin is quite delicate in this area, but gentler essential oils can reduce any of these troubling developments when used regularly. Here are some recipes for your eyes. Keep in mind these important tips: (1) Any sort of weight under the eyes pulls on the skin; always use a light amount. (2) Dab oil around the eye only, not the eyelids. (3) If you get any essential oil in the eye itself, immediately flush it out with lots of water.

- *Nighttime blend*
  Two teaspoons hazelnut oil
  Three drops evening primrose oil
  Two drops lavender essential oil
  One drop sandalwood essential oil
  Three drops carrot oil
  One capsule vitamin E (250 international units)

How to use: Mix the ingredients together, breaking open the vitamin E capsule but being careful not to touch the contents. Use a light amount around the eye. Leave the oil on for a few minutes, then gently dab off the excess. Use it nightly. As women mature, adding a second vitamin E capsule is recommended.

- *Puffiness/dark bags blend*
  Two teaspoons hazelnut oil
  One tablespoon witch hazel
  Two drops grapefruit essential oil
  Two drops chamomile

How to use: This recipe is a bit more complicated than most in my Natural Health and Beauty plan, but worth the effort if

Tea Break

Green tea is getting lots of praise from researchers for protecting against heart disease and some forms of cancer. It can also be a big boost for tired and saggy eyes. Keep a container of it cooled in the refrigerator, then dab around the eyes whenever you feel the peepers need a pick-me-up. Rosehips tea works, too.

your eyes are frequently puffy or dark bags are what you see every day in the mirror. The recipe starts with refrigerated witch hazel. Dissolve the grapefruit and chamomile oils into it and put it back in the fridge. Then wrap an ice cube in cotton gauze, dip it into the witch hazel–essential oils mixture and place it on the puffy or baggy area. Keep your eyes closed. Leave the cube in place for ten to fifteen seconds, then apply a small quantity of hazelnut oil while the area is still wet.

Lips Seal the Deal

There is no ignoring dry, cracked, chapped, or itchy lips. It has to be the top might-not-kill-you-but-sure-to-drive-you-crazy condition. The only things that rival it might be cold sores and canker sores. Essential oils can come to the rescue of your lips—and maybe your kissing habits along with it! Here are some ideas for chapped and sore lips, cold sores, canker sores, and herpes breakouts. This is one case in which I don't recommend sharing an *Earth Tribe* product with others in your family or circle of friends. Get enough *Earth Tribe Happy Chap* to go around!

- For chapped/sore lips and preventive maintenance: Use *Earth Tribe Happy Chap* with vitamins A, D, and E, plus the essential oil of orange. Its beeswax and soya oil base is easy on the lips while the oils are gentle but potent. Apply as necessary.

- For cold sores: Apply two to four drops of tea tree essential oil directly to lips with a cotton swab three to four times daily. Whenever you feel a breakout, start the treatment.

- For canker sores: Apply two to three drops of tea tree or lavender essential oils directly to infected area with a cotton swab two to three times daily.

- For herpes cold sores: Make this blend and apply it as necessary. If it seems to make the itchiness or tingling worse, try it without the bergamot.
  Eight drops geranium essential oil
  Three drops bergamot essential oil
  Six drops chamomile essential oil
  Eight drops tea tree essential oil
  Five drops lavender essential oil

Say Ah: Teeth and Gums

Oral hygiene is about more than avoiding bad breath or the dentist's chair. Research funded by the National Institutes of Health shows that people with more gum disease than others in the study also had more thickening of the arteries, which can lead to heart disease and stroke. Theories about why the cardiovascular system is affected by oral health include bacterial and viral infections moving through the bloodstream or causing inflammation of the arteries. More research is needed to make the direct link between gum problems and bigger problems, but why not take advantage of the antibacterial and antiviral properties of essential oils?

Here are some ideas for tooth and gum care to augment the normal brushing and flossing routine:

- General hygiene: Add two drops of peppermint, tea tree, lemon, or lavender essential oils to your toothpaste on the toothbrush. Soak your floss in a teaspoon of peppermint, tea tree, lemon, or lavender essential oils. Allow it to dry before using. Twice daily, use a mouthwash of two drops of peppermint essential oil and two drops of tea tree essential oil in a large glass of water. Swish well but do not swallow.

- Gum infections: Place two drops of tea tree oil on a cotton swab and rub gently over sore areas. Use the mouthwash described above.

- Toothache: Apply two drops of clove oil directly on affected area. You can substitute tea tree oil for lesser pain; clove oil is quite potent.

Fragrance: Less Is More

My stance on perfumes and body fragrances is straightforward. Don't use a lot of it, and use only the natural stuff. Throughout this book and my Healthy Living plan, I have emphasized the yin-yang type combination of gentleness and potency that is in every drop of essential oil. There's no reason to stop my mantra now!

Geranium as a single-note oil is wonderful for attracting others and, most important, gathering female energy. Wear a drop each on your pulse points. Patchouli is a basic ingredient of many classic erogenous perfumes. Bergamot lifts the spirits—yours and the people close to you. Lavender ranks high among the most pleasant smells for both men and women.

True essential oils possess bioelectrical energy, which they transfer to us in the form of an inner and outer *glow*. My take on synthetic fragrances and perfumes: they have a negative bio-electricity, they actually deplete our inner and outer *glow*. They drain life force from us.

Of course, I wholeheartedly recommend the *Earth Tribe Love* blend featuring ylang ylang and rose essential oils as an enchanting perfume. Rose essential oil worked for Cleopatra, it can work for us! While you are at it, add the *Love* blend to a diffuser in your bedroom. Sandalwood is a good single-note for romance and, please, use the *Earth Tribe*

Night Fire blend (ylang ylang and clove) in diffuser at your own risk—of losing sleep!

Romance can truly be in the air with essential oils. Just keep in mind less is more. Every small step counts for a lot.

Comparison Shopping

Here are some typical beauty categories and how *Earth Tribe* products can fill a need while eliminating chemicals from your daily life—and bathroom cabinet. *Earth Tribe* products are compared to what might be considered more natural product lines, so suffice it to say that the more popular brands of mass-produced, unabashedly artificial beauty and personal care products should already be in your wastebasket!

Mineral Baths/Bath Oils

Instead of using . . .

- The Village Bath Aromatic Bath Tablet

Try this alternative . . .

- *Earth Tribe Mint Salt Glow*

Instead of using . . .

- Clinique Body Scrub
- Lancôme Exfoliating Fraichelle

Try this alternative . . .

- *Earth Tribe Citrus Salt Glow*

Instead of using . . .
- Jean Naté Bath Oils
- Biotherm Body/Bath Oils

Try these alternatives . . .
- *Calming Body Oil*
- *Nightfire Body Oil*
- *Muscle Soothe Body Oil*

How to use: Place about one or two tablespoons of body/bath oils in the bath. Relax and soak.

Body Moisturizers/Slimming Lotions

Instead of using . . .
- Biotherm's Minceur Total

Try this alternative . . .
- *Earth Tribe Slim-u-lite*

How to use: Apply once or twice daily to hips, legs, abdomen, and upper arms after showering or bathing.

Bust Treatments

Instead of using . . .
- Lancôme's Energie Bust

Try this alternative . . .

- *Earth Tribe Cleavage Oil*

How to use: Massage on breast area twice daily to help improve circulation and enhance your skin's tone and texture.

Circulation/Tired, Sore Feet, and Legs

Instead of using . . .

- Body Shop Peppermint Foot Lotion

Try this alternative . . .

- *Earth Tribe Rejuvenator*

How to use: Apply to tired legs and feet morning and night, or as needed.

Facial Toners

Instead of using . . .

- Clinique Clarifying Lotion

Try this alternative . . .

- *Earth Tribe Plant Essence Skin Tonic*

How to use: Apply twice daily after cleansing to clear spent surface cells, make skin more receptive to moisture, reduce puffiness, and improve circulation. Contains grapefruit essential oils, which contain natural alpha hydroxy fruit acids.

Facial Moisturizers

Instead of using . . .

- Lancôme's Primordiale

Try this alternative . . .

- *Earth Tribe Ritual Beauty Potions Balancing Infusion No.1*

Instead of using . . .

- Origins Solutions

Try this alternative . . .

- *Earth Tribe Ritual Beauty Potions Balancing Infusion No.2*

How to use: Apply to entire face and neck twice daily after using facial toner. This formula contains rare, naturally occurring palmitoleic fatty acids found in our skin that tend to be lost as we age. You will find the product much lighter on the skin than lotions and creams, but it more easily penetrates the skin without clogging pores. *No. 1* is for dry to normal skin; *No. 2* is for oily skin.

Lip Balms

Instead of using . . .

- Body Shop lip balm

Try this alternative . . .

- *Earth Tribe Happy Chap*

How to use: Apply to lips as needed to moisturize and soothe dryness without artificial ingredients. Our all-natural, aromatic lip moisturizer contains only soya oil, beeswax, and vitamins A, D, and E, plus the essential oil of orange. It is a simple, effective formula that moisturizes and soothes dry or chapped lips without the unnecessary artificial ingredients.

Face/Body Cleansers

Instead of using . . .

- Clinique Facial Soap

Try these alternatives . . .

- *Earth Tribe Tea Tree Face Wash*
- *Earth Tribe Rose Geranium Face Wash*
- *Earth Tribe Helichrysum/Chamomile Face Wash*

Instead of using . . .

- Clarins Cleansing Gel

Try this alternative . . .

- *Earth Tribe Spirits Bath Gels*

How to use: *Tea Tree Face Wash* is restorative and gentle as the lead item on your beauty checklist. It clears the pores and repairs damage from facing the elements. It has antibacterial, antiviral, and antifungal properties for triple-threat protection. *Earth Tribe Spirits Bath Gels* are something completely different for consumers: They contain none of the harsh synthetic detergents found in almost all cleansing gels. Among the harsh chemicals: sodium lauryl sulfate, sodium laureth sulfate, and TEA and DEA sulfate. These gels come in three "flavors": *Euphoric Spirit Bath Gel* features bergamot and orange essential oils, *Calming Spirit Bath Gel* has lavender and chamomile, and *Refreshing Spirit Bath Gel* is a great wakeup blend of eucalyptus, lemon, geranium, and rosemary. Your skin becomes smooth, soft and silky—you will notice the difference.

Hair Care

Instead of using . . .

- All salon shampoos and conditioners

Try this alternative . . .

- *Earth Tribe Pure Botanical Shampoo & Conditioner*

How to use: Shampoo and condition hair daily if desired or as needed. *Earth Tribe Pure Botanical Shampoo* contains none of the synthetic detergents found in commercial shampoos, especially those used in salons and even products claiming to be all-natural. It took years to develop just the right formula that washes and revitalizes hair gently but effectively.

Cold and Flu Remedies

Instead of using . . .

- Tylenol Cold and Flu
- Afrin Nasal Spray

Try this alternative . . .

- *Earth Tribe Breathe*

How to use: For children, place a few drops in a room humidifier at night or place a few drops on the pillowcase or a favorite stuffed animal at night. During the day, place three drops of *Breathe* (you can substitute single-note eucalyptus) into one tablespoon of vegetable or nut oil. Rub the mixture on the chest. For adults, same routine as above but also feel free to put a couple of drops on your fingers to rub over your nose and up your forehead.

Aromatherapy Rubs

Instead of using . . .

- Vick's VapoRub

Try this alternative . . .

- *Earth Tribe Cold and Flu Rub*

How to use: Rub on your chest, neck, and back at the first sign of sickness. Safe for children but still effective for adults. One of *Earth Tribe's* most popular products and a true crowd-pleaser with parents.

First-Aid Skin Creams

Instead of using . . .

- Neosporin
- Desitin

Try this alternative . . .

- *Earth Tribe Herbal Comfort Cream*

How to use: Apply topically as needed. The therapeutic properties of the herb calendula and essential oils of lavender, tea tree, and chamomile combine to make an effective healing treatment for cuts, scrapes, rashes, burns, sunburn, dry and chapped skin, diaper rash, infections, and insect bites.

Headache Pain Relief

Instead of using . . .

- Excedrin
- Advil
- Tylenol

Try this alternative . . .

- *Earth Tribe Head Peace*

How to use: For headaches and migraine pain, put a couple of drops onto your fingertips and run into your temples and forehead and at the base of the skull, or wherever pain is located. Can also help relieve stress during times of intense mental concentration, and help you focus. Use sparingly, as this blend is very concentrated.

Instead of using . . .

- Motrin
- Midol

Try these alternatives . . .

- *Earth Tribe PMS Relief*
- *Earth Tribe Tummy Tonic*

How to use: Apply to the lower abdomen and lower back every hour as needed. Helps relieve discomfort quickly, safely, and naturally.

Muscle Aches

Instead of using . . .

- Bengay
- IcyHot

Try this alternative . . .

- *Earth Tribe Herbal Cooling Cream*

How to use: When feeling soreness, stiffness, or minor pain from athletics or physical activities, use as a soothing ointment. The cream feels good when you first apply it, and the healing effect will last longer than conventional ointments.

Instead of using . . .

- Aspercreme

Try this alternative . . .

- *Earth Tribe Muscle Soothe Essential Oil Blend*

How to use: For smaller areas of pain, such as wrists, fingers, ankles, shoulders, knees, and base of neck, apply topically as needed.

Earth Healing

Andreas Zafiriadis

Salon Buzz in Chicago lives up to its name. It is a super-busy place. In just a few years it has become Chicago's hippest place to get your hair styled. That doesn't stop owner and stylist Andreas Zafiriadis—the biggest reason why Salon Buzz is so hot and in high demand for world-class fashion shows—from looking for ways to help his customers relax while they're getting their hair styled, nails done, or a facial applied. He diffuses lavender and tangerine essential oils throughout his salon and plans to start adding essential oils to the shampoos and conditioners used in the salon. He is looking at installing an environmental fragrancing system, which makes him a visionary of sorts.

"I love lavender," says Andreas. "I truly believe essential oils have a direct link to our brains. I want our customers to be served to the fullest. The essential oils help us complete the experience. If I can figure out how to scent the whole salon more effectively but without disturbing or distracting the customers in any way, we'll do it. We always want to be on the cutting edge."

What's more, Andreas uses lavender at home. His upstairs diffusers rarely go without it. "Our home is my place to unwind and kick back," says Andreas. "The lavender sets the mood right away when I walk in the door."

Safety Information

General precautions:

- As with any concentrated substance, you'll want to keep essential oils out of the reach of children and away from pets. Do not take any oils by mouth.
- Because of the potency of essential oils, proceed carefully and with guidance from a health professional if you have any of the following conditions: pregnancy (see Pregnancy Pause in Chapter 9 for more details, plus the listing below), high blood pressure, epilepsy, open wounds, diabetes, rashes, or neurological disorders; or if you are taking prescribed medications and/or homeopathic remedies.

- These oils are not intended to replace medical treatment. You should seek diagnosis and recommendations from a licensed health practitioner for serious medical concerns. I do not intend to prescribe or diagnose.
- Do not apply photosensitive essential oils, including bergamot, orange, lemon, and grapefruit, to the skin. Avoid skin contact with peppermint and rosemary essential oils.
- Avoid juniper essential oil if you have kidney disease. Avoid rosemary essential oil if you have high blood pressure or a seizure disorder. Avoid *Earth Tribe Even Tides, Slim Scents,* and *Energize* essential oil blends if you have a seizure disorder.

The do's and don'ts of essential oils during pregnancy:

- Avoid these essential oils entirely during pregnancy: rosemary, juniper, *Earth Tribe Head Peace, Energize, Even Tides, Tummy Tonic, Sweet Dreams, Slim-u-lite, Mint Salt Glow, PMS Relief Rub, Prosperity,* and *Slim Scents* blends. During the first three months of pregnancy, the body is doing a great job—and knows how to do it quite well. I recommend using only lavender essential oil, *Earth Tribe Mother and Baby Massage Oil, Calming Massage Oil,* or *Calming* blend during this time.
- Please see Pregnancy Pause in Chapter 9 for more detailed information.

Appendix A

Earth Tribe Essential Oils and Products

Here is a convenient listing of the essential oils and related products sold by my company, Earth Tribe. For more information, call 800-8TRIBE8, or 800-887-4238. You can also visit our Internet site at www.earth-tribe.com.

Single Notes
- ### Bergamot

Cheerful and uplifting, often used in European clinics to treat depression. Also used for anxiety/stress relief, mind-body balance, to curb mood swings, and as an immune system booster. Part of the citrus fruit family.

• **Eucalyptus**

Cools the body in summer and protects it in winter. Used as a disinfectant, an insect repellant, a decongestant, for relief from sinus pain and sore muscles, to reduce acne/blemishes, and to promote mind-body balance.

• **Geranium**

Wonderful worn alone as a perfume and extremely uplifting. Works well for female energy. Also good for relief from anxiety/stress, depression, menopause symptoms, and PMS. It also normalizes dry or oily skin and promotes hormonal balance.

• **Grapefruit**

Terrific oil for the kitchen. Helps eliminate odors and cuts grease. Acts as an astringent and facial toner. Also used for cellulite, lymphatic drainage, and water retention.

• **Juniper**

Highly rejuvenating in the bath. Helps reduce water retention. Acts as an astringent and toxin eliminator. Energizing and invigorating.

• **Lavender**

The most gentle and versatile oil, as we learned in Chapter 1. Excellent for children's and infants' baths. Highly calming. Also used to treat blemishes, burns, insomnia, nervous tension, rashes, scrapes/cuts, and sunburn.

• **Lemon**

Carries solar vitality to the body, mind, and soul. Think of it as the sun's golden gift. Refreshes and revives, disinfects, but remember never to use directly on skin without diluting by carrier oil. Used for stress relief, depression, and cold and flu symptoms.

• Orange

Great scent for kids. Ideal in the kitchen as a freshener. Can be an effective insect repellant. Used for depression, lymphatic drainage, and to decrease wrinkles.

• Patchouli

Basic ingredient of many classic erogenous perfumes. Works as an aphrodisiac. Helps you feel grounded. Also used to balance emotions, soothe dry skin, and repel insects.

• Peppermint

Cooling after a workout or other strenuous activity. Use with base oil as an after-workout spray or add some drops to your bath or shower. Also used to help with muscle pain, digestive problems, bad breath, and headaches.

• Rose

The symbol for love, sensuality, and compassion. Helps release anger and grief. Works as an antiseptic and infection fighter. Used to help with PMS discomfort and insomnia, to encourage cell rejuvenation, and to heal eczema and broken capillaries. The most precious (and expensive) among common essential oils.

• Rosemary

Protective scent that helps clear negative energy from one's aura and environment. Energizing. Effective in treating headaches and promoting mental concentration and enhancing memory.

• Sandalwood

Woodsy, earthy scent offers meditative qualities. Can be used as an aphrodisiac and sexual restorative for men and women. Other applications include as an appetite depressant, a sedative, and a stress reliever. More expensive than most oils.

- Tea tree

Currently one of the most studied essential oils because it can help treat both bacterial and viral infections, plus athlete's foot, acne, cold sores, gum problems, flu symptoms, insect bites, rashes, and yeast infections. A must item for the medicine cabinet.

Synergistic Essential Oil Blends
- Balance

This blend is the natural solution to the ups and downs of every day life. Essential oils have been confirmed as effective antidepressants that will balance moods and emotions. Main ingredients: rose and bergamot.

- Breathe

A blend of oils carefully formulated to help relieve colds, congestion, sinusitis, and coughs. Main ingredients: eucalyptus and fir balsam.

- Calming

A wonderful formulation that helps to melt stress, plus induce feelings of tranquility and serenity. Main ingredients: lavender and chamomile.

- Courage

Inspired by a Native American tradition in which cedar and pine boughs were rubbed on the body to promote inner strength and purity, and to ground emotions. Pine has been considered the *cleansing oil* for centuries. Main ingredients: spruce and cedarwood.

- Detox

This blend is formulated with essential plant oils that aid the body in eliminating toxins and stubborn fatty deposits. Also very helpful for a body that retains water. Main ingredients: juniper, grapefruit, and fennel.

• Energize

Jump-start your mornings and your workouts, or relieve afternoon energy lows and general fatigue with this stimulating blend. Main ingredients: juniper and peppermint.

• Euphoria

A formulation of the oils traditionally known to carry euphoric qualities. Euphoria helps to promote joy, playfulness, and a sense of well-being. Main ingredients: orange and bergamot.

• Even Tides

A comforting and balancing formulation specifically designed to help alleviate the uncomfortable symptoms of PMS and menopause. Strengthens and supports female energy. Main ingredients: clary sage and sweet fennel.

• Head Peace

A powerful blend of oils designed to help ease the pain of headaches and migraines, and enhance mental clarity, focus, and vision. Main ingredients: basil and rosemary.

• Love

A very romantic blend, formulated with oils that have symbolized and enhanced love throughout time. Makes an enchanting perfume! Main ingredients: ylang ylang and rose.

• Muscle Soothe

A soothing formulation designed to help alleviate the discomforts of overworked, overstressed muscles, strains and sprains, sore muscles, and joints. Main ingredients: sweet birch and peppermint.

• Night Fire

A provocative combination of nature's aphrodisiacs used for centuries to entice and captivate. This mysterious blend truly sets the mood. Main ingredients: ylang ylang and clove.

• Prosperity

A very special blend of oils that in ancient times were considered more valuable than gold. Based on time-honored tradition, this formula is designed to bring prosperity in health, wealth, family, and love. Main ingredients: frankincense and myrrh.

• Recovery

Balancing and stabilizing, this carefully formulated blend supports a balanced connection to earth, aligning body, mind, and spirit. It is especially healing to the joints, providing relief to anyone with arthritis symptoms. Helps to retain one's unique powers by recovering positive emotions and grounding the self. Balances male energy. Main ingredients: vetiver and cedarwood.

• Sweet Dreams

For restless nights and general insomnia, keep this blend close at hand. A combination of very sedating oils that help to bring on a deep, restful sleep. Main ingredients: marjoram and lavender.

• Tummy Tonic

A tummy rub to help alleviate the discomfort of upset stomachs caused by travel, nerves, flu, and overindulging! Main ingredients: peppermint and ginger.

•Volupte

Earth Tribe's first exotic perfume blend made with 100 percent pure and natural essential oils. As the name implies, this rich blend of rare and precious oils creates a sensuous and pleasurable mood, at the same time promoting a delightfully soothing, warm feeling. Main ingredients: rose, jasmine, and frankincense.

Essential Oil Health Boosters

• Herbal Comfort Cream

An effective healing treatment for rashes, cuts, scrapes, burns, diaper rash, dry or chapped skin, sunburn, insect bites, and eczema. One of our natural salves that every home should have on hand. Main ingredients: lavender, tea tree and chamomile essential oils, the herb calendula.

• Herbal Cooling Cream

A highly effective, soothing ointment for muscle soreness, athletic injuries, strains and sprains, back pain, tired aching muscles, and insect bites. Main ingredients: peppermint, lavender, and birch essential oils; the herb, St. John's wort, and aloe vera.

• Cold and Flu Rub

Utilizing nature's most potent ingredients, this traditional remedy rub helps to fortify the body while releasing toxins and easing the discomforts of cold and flu. It serves as triple threat of antibacterial, antiviral, and antifungal. Apply topically; for children and adults. Main ingredients: lavender, tea tree, manuka, and eucalyptus essential oils.

• PMS Relief Rub

This skillfully crafted formula, when applied over the lower abdomen and lower back, helps to relieve pain and discomfort associated with premenstrual syndrome. The balancing scent also helps lift the spirits. Main ingredients: peppermint, marjoram, and clary sage essential oils.

Face and Body Care

Each "Balancing Infusion" face oil is formulated for a certain skin type, as outlined here. All of them contain the rare macadamia nut oil, which most closely represents the oils of our skin.

• Balancing Infusion No. 1

Designed for dry/mature skin with the cell regenerating benefits of lavender and frankincense essential oils and the balancing effects of rose and geranium. Tip: If your skin is extremely dry, add two to three drops of sandalwood to the face oil when applying it to your face.

• Balancing Infusion No. 2

Formulated for normal/oily skin, with the antibacterial properties of tea tree and eucalyptus essential oils and the soothing effects of lavender.

• Balancing Infusion No. 3

For sensitive skin that has tendencies toward dryness. Its Roman chamomile and sandalwood essential oils quickly calm and restore the natural balance of the skin, while the lavender and evening primrose oils aid in cellular rejuvenation.

• Balancing Infusion No. 4

Carefully crafted for problem skin, such as rosacea, acne, and blemished skin. This unique infusion contains healing helichrysum and chamomile manuka, which work to quickly calm, clear, and balance the skin.

• Cleavage Oil

The breast area needs special care, and European women have long used and sworn by the "phyto-hormone" rich plant essences contained in this formulation. Massage on breast area twice daily to help moisturize and improve circulation, enhancing the skin's texture and tone. It features a blend of geranium, rose, lavender, clary sage, and fennel essential oils.

- **Rejuvenator Massage Oil**

A unique blend of cypress, peppermint, and marjoram essential oils helps to improve circulation, while supporting the elimination of toxins in joints and tissues. Amazingly soothing and rejuvenating for tired and swollen feet and legs, as well as other areas of the body.

- **Plant Essence Skin Tonic**

This amazing skin tonic leaves your skin feeling naturally clean and fresh. It improves circulation, reduces puffiness, tightens pores, and firms skin. Contains a unique combination of pure plant and flower essences, including a rare fluid extract of witch hazel without alcohol. Features a power-packed essential oils blend of cypress, lavender, juniper, grapefruit, and orange.

- **Citrus Salt Glow**

A refreshing gentle full-body exfoliation designed to whisk away dead skin cells and gently detoxify the tissues to reveal softer, healthy looking skin. Use even where skin is driest. Its main ingredients are sea salts, plus essential oils of orange, lemon, and tangerine.

- **Invigorating Mint Salt Glow**

A rejuvenating full-body exfoliation designed to whisk away dead skin cells and gently detoxify the tissues to reveal softer-looking skin. A fantastic wake-up call for the body and mind in the morning! Sea salts combined with essential oils of peppermint, mint, geranium, and eucalyptus.

- **Calming Spirit Bath Gel**

One of our line of all-natural bath and shower gels with no harsh synthetic chemicals and other artificial ingredients. *Calming Spirit Bath Gel* is a perfect cleanser for nighttime bathing and any time you need to de-stress. Features the essential oils of lavender and chamomile in *Earth Tribe's Calming* synergistic blend.

• Euphoric Spirit Bath Gel

A 100 percent natural bath gel that will lift your spirits morning or evening. Features the essential oils of orange and bergamot in *Earth Tribe's Euphoric* synergistic blend.

• Refreshing Spirit Bath Gel

This bath gel can serve as your everyday soap rather than products with synthetic chemicals. An all-natural combination that features the essential oils of eucalyptus, geranium, lemon, and rosemary.

• Tea Tree Face Wash

An all-natural face wash without any of the harsh synthetic chemicals of typical face cleansers. You will be converted after a day or two of washing! The main ingredients are tea tree and lavender essential oils.

• Pure Botanical Formula Shampoo

Earth Tribe's pure natural botanical shampoo is formulated with nature's most effective flower and herb extracts to naturally clean and revitalize hair. One big advantage of *Earth Tribe* shampoo compared to commercial brands with synthetic chemicals is the success of essential oils in restoring hair's natural balance of oils. Your hair doesn't get too dry or too oily. Features a hair-healthy combination of rosemary, lavender, sandalwood, and tea tree essential oils, plus aloe vera.

• Rose Geranium Face Wash

Our all natural face wash suitable for drier skin.

- **Helichrysum/Chamomile Deep Healing Face Wash**

A deep-healing, effective, and gentle face wash for all skin types that works especially well on acne and rosacea.

- **Pure Botanical Formula Conditioner**

Earth Tribe's pure natural botanical creme conditioner is formulated with rosemary, lavender, sandalwood, and tea tree essential oils and aloe vera. Protects against frizzing, splitting and other "bad hair" features. Like a spa treatment for your hair!

Home and Garden
- **All-Natural Insect Repellant**

Based on plant oils used by Native Americans for centuries to keep mosquitoes, flies, ticks, even ants away. This blend of orange, peppermint, cedarwood, lemon, lavender, and patchouli essential oils is extremely effective, but safe and gentle enough for your entire family. It is also a wonderful skin moisturizer.

- **Claire**

Use this organic, plant oil based antiseptic spray anytime, anywhere to clean, disinfect and freshen naturally. More effective than harsh synthetic commercial brands, yet 100 percent natural and nontoxic. Features a powerful blend of lavender, lemon, orange, eucalyptus, and tea tree essential oils. Gentle enough for use on the body to quickly clean and freshen.

Massage Oils/Body Oils
- **Mother and Baby Massage Oil**

A soothing all-over body moisturizer. Use throughout your pregnancy to keep skin smooth and soft, and to help in preventing stretch marks. Keep this blend on hand for the new baby, as it also makes a gentle, calming massage for baby. Main ingredients: lavender and chamomile.

• Slim-u-lite Body Oil

Quickly becoming a favorite, this blend is formulated with four essential plant oils that aid the body in breaking down stubborn fatty deposits and getting rid of excess water. Leaves the skin silky soft. Main ingredients: cypress, juniper, grapefruit, and fennel.

• Muscle Soothe Body Oil

Relax and relieve discomfort in sore, tired muscles before or after strenuous activity. A great all-over body massage for the active. Main ingredients: peppermint and sweet birch.

• Calming Body Oil

A bestseller with massage therapists and parents! This relaxing massage oil is the perfect rubdown for overworked, overstressed adults; a terrific rub for calming little ones! Main ingredients: lavender, sandalwood, tangerine.

• Night Fire Body Oil

A highly sensual massage, bath, or body oil, this provocative formulation utilizes nature's most effective aphrodisiacs to help set the mood. Main ingredients: sandalwood, patchouli, and clove.

• Volupte Body Oil

This luxurious body oil has been created with rare and precious pure essential oils which pamper your body and soul. Delight in the sensuous and pleasurable feelings of this blend. Main ingredients: sandalwood, jasmine, and rose.

Tribe Kids

• Monster Mist

This spray bottle (the perfect size for little hands to grasp) is filled with a *magical* formula that repels monsters and ghouls of all sorts when sprayed by a child throughout his or her room. The "magical" formula is actually a carefully chosen blend of essential oils clinically proven to calm, pacify, and comfort—while purifying and cleansing the air—100 percent natural and nontoxic!

Directions: Have child spray the bedroom or sleeping area with the *Monster Mist* to keep monsters at bay, and to aid in calming and helping to sleep.

Ingredients: pure spring water, essential oils of Bulgarian lavender, Roman chamomile, and sweet orange.

•Owie Juice

A spray bottle with a blend of essential oils that disinfect, relieve pain and promote the healing process (cell rejuvenation) for first-aid needs: cuts, scrapes, burns, insect bites, bruises, sunburn. This formula is perfectly safe for topical applications without any side effects.

Directions: Spray on topically as needed.

Ingredients: pure spring water, powdered honey, aloe vera juice, essential oils of Bulgarian lavender, Australian tea tree, and Roman chamomile.

•Lullabye Baby Rub

This gentle baby oil is formulated with a blend of essential oils that help comfort, calm, and soothe babies when gently massaged. It works especially well when massaged on the tummy area for colic. Can also be used as a bath oil.

Directions: Gently massage on baby; for colicky babies, gently massage over the tummy area. As a bath oil, place a small amount (1 tsp.) in baby's bath.

Ingredients: grapeseed oil, soybean oil, essential oils of Bulgarian lavender, Roman chamomile, and dill.

• Baby Balm

A natural alternative to commercial diaper rash ointments that contain harsh synthetic chemicals. The perfect, natural solution for diaper rash, cradle cap, or any of the minor skin irritations that babies sometimes get.

Directions: Apply topically to baby's skin as needed.

Ingredients: pure beeswax, soybean oil, calendula oil, aloe vera juice and essential oils of Bulgarian lavender, Australian tea tree, and Roman chamomile.

• Happy Chap

This gentle, 100 percent natural lip balm is made with plant oils that have an aromatherapeutic effect of promoting joy and happiness. Very soothing and nourishing for dry, cracked lips. Comes in an easy-to-apply tube.

Directions: Apply topically on lips as needed.

Ingredients: pure beeswax, soybean oil, and essential oil of sweet orange.

• Pure Botanical Baby Shampoo & Bath Gel

This completely natural and gentle *no tears* antibacterial shampoo and bath gel is made without the harsh synthetic detergents found in most baby shampoos and bath gels. Excellent for babies' skin, including cradle cap.

Directions: Pour a small amount into hands, then gently massage into a lather on baby's hair and rinse. As a bath gel, use in bath to cleanse body, or for a natural bubble bath, pour under faucet as you run the bath.

Ingredients: purified water, aloe vera gel, coconut oil olefin, coconut oil betaine, avocado oil, lemon extract, essential oils of Australian tea tree and Bulgarian lavender, and vitamins A, C, and E.

Envrionmental Fragrancing

• Moon and Star Aroma Lamp

Through the delicate union of ancient tradition and modern technology, aroma lamps bring natural environmental fragrancing to your home. They are perfect for larger rooms. There is no candle, simply a low-watt lightbulb that heats the oils gently and slowly diffuses them into the air. Fill the built-in bowl with clean water, add six to twelve drops of your favorite essential or blend, and enjoy!

•Clay Pot Diffuser

These pottery diffusers are just right for smaller rooms—as well as your automobiles and office cubicles. Put twenty to thirty drops of an essential oil or blend directly into the top of the bottle. The oils diffuse slowly through the terra-cotta, which is only glazed on the bottom. Get several for your personal spaces.

•Terra-cotta Lightbulb Rings

Place your lightbulb ring atop a standard lightbulb. Add eight to twelve drops of essential oil or blend to the inner rim. The room will quickly fill with natural fragrance.

•Earth Tribe Base Spray

Our all-natural, water-soluble *Earth Tribe Base Spray* facilitates the use of essential oils and blends as a room spray/air freshener or body spray. Place thirty to fifty drops of essential oil or blend into the *Base Spray*. Shake well and spray your environment (home, office, car, etc.) or yourself. A natural way to disinfect the air.

•Nebulizing Diffuser

For maximum therapeutic effect, I recommend the nebulizing diffuser. When essential oils are diffused through a nebulizer, they are broken down into extremely tiny particles that stay suspended in your environment for an extended period. Each time you inhale, your lungs and other organs—in fact all of your cells—are drawing in the benefits of essential oils.

Appendix B

Suggested Reading and Reference List

Here is a list of books, journal articles, Internet sites, research organizations, government agencies, and other sources used to write this book. Many of the sources are valuable for learning more about specific essential oils or aromatherapy as a healing practice. Some references noted also apply to subsequent chapters.

Introduction

Eisenberg, D., et al. "Trends in Alternative Medicine Use in the United States, 1990–1997: Results of a Follow-up National Survey," *Journal of the American Medical Association*, 280 (1998), pp. 1569–75.

Chapter 1

Blumenthal, M., J. Gruenwald, T. Hall, and R. S. Rister, eds. *The Complete German Commission E Monographs: Therapeutic Guide to Herbal Medicine*. Boston: Integrative Medicine Communications, 1998.

Buchbauer, G., et al. "Aromatherapy: Evidence for Sedative Effects of the Essential Oil of Lavender after Inhalation," *Nature*, 16 (1991), pp. 1067–72.

Cornwell, Dale A. and S., "The Role of Lavender Oil in Relieving Perineal Discomfort Following Childbirth: A Blind Randomized Trial," *Journal of Advanced Nursing*, 19 (1994), pp. 89–96.

Hardy, M., et al. "Replacement of Drug Therapy for Insomnia by Ambient Odour," *The Lancet*, 346 (Sept. 9, 1995), p. 701.

Mailhebiau, Phillipe. *Portraits in Oils: The Personality of Aromatherapy Oils and Their Link with Human Temperaments* (abridged version of *La Nouvelle Aromathérapie* by Mailhebiau). C. W. Daniel, 1995.

Pattnaik, S., et al. "Antibacterial and Antifungal Activity of Aromatic Constituents of Essential Oils," *Microbiology*, 89 (1997), pp. 39–46.

Chapter 2

Jacob, S., et al. "Location and Gross Morphology of the Nasopalatine Duct in Human Adults," *Archives of Otolaryngology-Head and Neck Surgery*, 126 (June 2000), pp. 741–48.

McClintock, M. "Regulation of Ovulation by Human Pheromones," *Nature*, 392 (March 12, 1998), pp. 177–79.

Valnet, Jean. *The Practice of Aromatherapy*. C. W. Daniel/Saffron Walden, 1982.

Chapter 3

Prochaska, James O. *Changing for Good*. Avon, 1995.

Taste and Small Laboratory, Duke University Medical Center, Durham, N.C., Susan Schiffman, director, www.duke.edu/~sss/tsi.html.

U.S. Environmental Protection Agency, Office of Prevention, Pesticides and Toxic Substances, www.epa.gov/opptsfrs/home/

Chapter 4

Lamberg, Lynne. *Bodyrhythms: Chronobiology and Peak Performance*. Morrow, 1994.

Chapter 5

Case, R. B., et al. "Living Alone After Myocardial Infarction: Impact on Prognosis," *Journal of the American Medical Association*, 267 (1991), pp. 515–19.

Devanand, D. P. "Olfactory Deficits in Patients with Mild Cognitive Impairment Predict Disease at Follow-up," *American Journal of Psychiatry*, 157 (Sept 2000), pp. 1399–1405.

Eliot, Dr. Robert S. *From Stress to Strength: How to Lighten Your Load and Save Your Life*. Bantam, 1995.

Katz, Lawrence C. *Keep Your Brain Alive: 83 Neurobic Exercises to Help Prevent Memory Loss and Increase Mental Fitness*. Workman, 1999.

Marmot, M.G., et al. "Employment Grade and Coronary Heart Disease in British Civil Servants," *Journal of Epidemiology and Community Health*, 3 (1978), pp. 244–49.

Monell Chemical Senses Center, Philadelphia, www.monell.org/sensation.htm.

Smell and Taste Treatment and Research Foundation, Chicago, Dr. Alan R. Hirsch, director, www.smellandtaste.org.

Williams, Virginia and Redford. *Life-Skills: 8 Simple Ways to Build Stronger Relationships, Communicate More Clearly and Improve Your Health and Even the Health of Those Around You.* Times Books, 1997.

Williams, R. B. "Prognostic Importance of Social and Economic Resources Among Medically Treated Patients with Angiographically Documented Coronary Artery Disease," *Journal of the American Medical Association,* 267 (1992), pp. 520–24.

Chapter 6

American Lung Association, www.lungusa.org.

American Society of Heating, Refrigerating and Air-Conditioning Engineers, *IAQ Applications* journal (Summer 2000), www.ashrae.org.

Consumer Product Safety Commission, www.cdsc.gov/library.

Dadd, Debra Lynn. *Home Safe Home: Protecting Yourself and Your Family from Everyday Toxics and Harmful Household Products.* Tarcher/Putnam, 1997.

U.S. Environmental Protection Agency. *Read the Label First! Protect Your Kids,* EPA Document No. 740-F-00-001. www.epa.gov or contact National Service Center for Environmental Publications, P.O. Box 42419, Cincinnati, OH 45242-0419 (513) 490-8190 or (800) 490-9198.

U.S. Environmental Protection Agency. *The Inside Story: A Guide to Indoor Air Quality,* EPA Document No. 402-K-93-007. www.epa.gov/iaq/pubs/insideest.html.

Chapter 7

"Be Smart About Using Antibiotics," *Dr. Andrew Weil's Self Healing* newsletter, Oct. 2000, pp. 2–3.

Institute of Food Technologists. Presentation at 1999 annual meeting, Daniel Y.C. Fung, Kansas State University. www.sciencedaily.com or www.ksu.edu.

Ott, W. R., and J. W. Roberts. "Everyday Exposure to Toxic Pollutants," *Scientific American,* Feb. 1998.

Sherman, P. "Antimicrobial Functions of Spices: Why Some Like It Hot," *Quarterly Review of Biology,* 73 (March 1998), pp. 3–49.

Weil, Dr. Andrew. *Spontaneous Healing: How to Discover and Enhance Your Body's Natural Ability to Maintain and Heal Itself.* Ballantine, 1995.

Chapter 8

Diego, M. A., et al. "Aromatherapy Reduces Anxiety and Enhances EEG Patterns Associated with Positive Mood and Alertness," *International Journal of Neuroscience,* 96 (1998), pp. 217–224.

Holmes, T. H., and R. H. Rahe. *Journal of the Psychosomatic Research,* 11 (1967), pp. 213–18.

"Stress Taking a Toll on Children's Health," *Chicago Tribune,* Sept. 24, 2000.

University of Wisconsin Health Emotions Research Institute, Dr. Ned Kalin, director, www.healthemotions.org.

Chapter 9

Armstrong, F. "Scenting Relief," *Nursing Times,* 87 (1991), pp. 52–54.

Benson, Herbert, and M. Kippler. *The Relaxation Response.* Avon, 1976.

Burns, E., et al. "The Use of Aromatherapy in Intrapartum Midwifery Practice," Oxford Centre for Health Care Research and Development/Oxford Brookes University, 1999, www.Brookes.ac.uk/h/ochrd/uaimp.html.

Field, T., et al. "Massage of Preterm Newborns to Improve Growth and Development," *Pediatric Nursing,* 13 (1987), pp. 385–87.

Field, T., et al. "Massage with Oil has More Positive Effects on Newborn Infants," *Pre and Perinatal Psychology Journal,* 11 (1996), pp. 73–78.

Field, T., et al. "Alleviating Posttraumatic Stress in Children Following Hurricane Andrew," *Journal of Applied Developmental Psychology,* 17 (1996), pp. 37–50.

Gump, B. B., and K. A. Matthews. "Are Vacations Good for Your Health? The 9-Year Mortality Experience After the Multiple Risk Factor Intervention Trial," *Psychosomatic Medicine,* 62 (Sept./Oct. 2000), pp. 608–12.

Hooper, P. L. "Hot-Tub Therapy for Type 2 Diabetes," *New England Journal of Medicine,* 34 (Sept. 16, 1999), pp. 924–25.

Murphy, P. and S. Campbell. "Nightime Drop in Body Temperature: A Physiological Trigger for Sleep Onset?" *Sleep,* 20 (1997), pp. 505–11.

National Sleep Foundation, www.sleepfoundation.org.

Ornish, Dean, *Dr. Dean Ornish's Program for Reversing Heart Disease.* Ballantine, 1990.

Prodromidis, M., T. Field, et al. "Mothers Touching Newborns: A Comparison of Rooming-in Versus Minimal Contact," *Birth*, 22 (1995), pp. 196–200.

Tattam, A. "The Gentle Touch," *Nursing Times*, 88 (1992), pp. 54–55.

Touch Research Institute, University of Miami School of Medicine, Dr. Tiffany Fields, director, www.miami.edu/touch-research/index.html.

Chapter 10

U.S. Food and Drug Administration, www.fda.gov (see "Soap"and "Cosmetics" categories). The Soap position paper is 1995; the Cosmetics position paper was originally done in 1998 and updated in 2000.

Chapter 11

"Gum Disease: Not Just a Pain in the Mouth," *Science Reporter,* May 6, 1998. www.heartinfo.org/science/gum5698.htm.

National Institute of Dental and Craniofacial Research, www.nidcr.nih.gov/news/al.htm.

About the Authors

MARY LEE PATTON is the founder and CEO of Earth Tribe International, a Santa Monica, California–based company that offers a full line of all-natural essential oil products for personal health and beauty care, children, household cleaning, pets, and much more. Mary Lee learned about natural healing and beauty secrets from her upbringing amid nature in northern Minnesota, and from studying essential oils and herbs throughout the United States and Europe. She is the mother of twin boys, who continually motivate her to find new ways to convince people to eliminate synthetic chemicals from their lives. She lives in Santa Monica and northern Minnesota with her husband, Jim, and her twin sons.

BOB CONDOR is the health and fitness columnist for the *Chicago Tribune*. His columns and stories appear in more than one hundred U.S. newspapers and Internet sites. He lives in Chicago with his wife, Mary, and their two young children.